The 5:2 bikini diet : over 140 ... help you los

JACQU ... WN

THE
5:2
BIKINI
DIET

Over 140 delicious recipes that
will help you lose weight, fast

HarperCollins*Publishers*

HarperCollins*Publishers*
77–85 Fulham Palace Road
London W6 8JB

www.harpercollins.co.uk

1 3 5 7 9 10 8 6 4 2

Text © Jacqueline Whitehart 2013

Exercise programme © Sculpt Health and Fitness Ltd

Jacqueline Whitehart asserts her moral right to be
identified as the author of this work.

Photography © Myles New 2013
Food stylist: Annie Hudson
Prop stylist: Lucy Harvey

Library of Congress Cataloging-in-Publication Data
available upon request.

PB ISBN: 978-0-00-723765-4
UK EB ISBN: 978-0-00-723766-1
US EB ISBN: 978-0-00-752822-8

Printed and bound in the United States of America by
RR Donnelley

This book features weight-loss techniques which may not be suitable for
everyone. You should always consult with a qualified medical practitioner
before starting any weight-loss programme, or if you have any concerns about
your health. This book is not tailored to individual requirements or needs
and its contents are solely for general information purposes. It should not be
taken as professional or medical advice or diagnosis. The activities detailed in
this book should not be used as a substitute for any treatment or medication
prescribed or recommended to you by a medical practitioner. The author
and the publishers do not accept any responsibility for any adverse effects
that may occur as a result of the use of the suggestions or information herein.
If you feel that you are experiencing adverse effects after embarking
on any weight-loss programme, including the type described in this
book, it is imperative that you seek medical advice. Results may
vary from individual to individual.

For my husband Andy who has helped and supported me both in life-style changes and in my writing. He has also enthusiastically tested out all my new recipes.

For my children Amy, Irie and Max who remind me that life isn't just a diet.

CONTENTS

PART 1

THE

5:2

BIKINI
DIET

INTRODUCTION

The 5:2 Bikini Diet has something to offer everyone as it's totally different to other diets – diet twice a week, then eat healthily the rest of the time and watch the weight fall off. As an avid follower of the 5:2 diet since September 2012, I want to share my experiences of this life- and figure-changing diet with the world.

I have created an all-new and delicious selection of healthy and filling recipes that are just perfect for summer. You will find salads, barbecues and super summer desserts, which are all suitable for your fast days.

With the addition of a simple and fun exercise routine, developed by David Jones of Sculpt Health & Fitness, this is the perfect diet to lose weight and get in shape for the summer.

This book is for you if you are new to the diet and want to get started; if you are already a follower of the 5:2 diet and are looking for some extra help or a new start; if you want some fantastic new recipes for summer; if you want an exercise routine that will improve your bikini body or you just want to lose some weight in a healthy and simple way.

Join the 5:2 revolution and be happy with your weight **and** your body. I'll see you on the beach!

Yours,

Jacqueline

Jacqueline Whitehart, April 2013

THE GOLDEN RULES FOR A SUCCESSFUL DIET

Let's cut to the chase: there are three steps that we will be following for the next four weeks and beyond to get into shape for the summer. Follow these rules and you will lose weight, feel healthier and look great.

- Fast – eat only 500 calories for women/600 calories for men – on two non-consecutive days per week.
- Eat normally but healthily on the other five days.
- Follow the 30-minute workout plan three times a week on your non-fasting days.

Looks simple doesn't it? That's because it is! It's really simple and easy to follow, so read on and I will guide you through each of the three rules.

1 Fast twice a week

Two days a week you follow a calorie-restricted diet, that's:
- 500 calories for women
- 600 calories for men

The days are non-consecutive.

2 Eat normally but healthily on the other five days

If you have followed the 5:2 diet before you will be familiar with the term 'feast' day, but that's something that trips people up time and time again. This is because most of us, if told we can eat what we like, go a bit mad.

The five non-fast days are normal and healthy days, they are not diet days and we do not count calories.

DO:
- Enjoy your food and don't count the calories.
- Eat three healthy meals a day.
- Do NOT snack between meals and avoid processed food.

Cut out the rubbish. Keep the following items to a very bare minimum:
- biscuits (cookies) and cakes
- crisps (potato chips)
- non-diet fizzy drinks
- chocolate bars and sweets (candies)
- beer, lager and cider

If you follow these steps, you will have plenty of scope for tasty plates of food without excluding any food group, and it means that you will be able to have delicious pasta, bread, desserts and, of course, a glass or two of wine.

Remember that the recipes in this book are not just for fast days; they are perfect for your normal days too. Just add some extra carbohydrates, such as rice or potatoes, if necessary and make sure you eat three balanced meals every day.

3 Exercise three times a week

While rules 1 and 2 are for weight loss, exercise makes the most of the weight loss by reducing the flab, toning your body and zapping the cellulite.

If you are new to exercise, then perhaps the best way to get started is walking. Start with walking 15 minutes a day, three days a week and work up from there. Walking is great if you are just starting to exercise as it is proven to significantly improve fitness levels. Walking increases the blood flow to the muscles, improving circulation and heart function.

Swimming is also a suitable option if you are just getting started with exercise.

If you are fit and exercise regularly then you should find Sculpt's 5:2 Bikini Diet exercise plan easy and enjoyable, ready to get your body in shape for the summer – fast!

By following the workout plan three times a week, you can expect great results in just four weeks. There's more detail about the benefits of combining exercise with the 5:2 diet in the 'Getting beach fit' chapter (see page 40).

HEALTH BENEFITS
Not just slimming

This chapter simply explains the medical reasons for the diet's success. When you understand how healthy you will become on this diet – as well as slimming easily – you will keep to this lifestyle forever. The slimming results on the 5:2 Bikini Diet are stunning. And not just that, losing weight healthily and easily improves your overall health. There is also increasing evidence that this new breed of fast diet, of which the 5:2 diet is the easiest and most popular, has some incredible benefits for your long-term health too.

What happens in our bodies when we fast?

Based on the opinion of several fasting experts, there is now a picture developing of how the scientists believe intermittent fasting changes the way our bodies work, giving us additional health benefits as we age. Here I provide a simple approach to the science, which I hope will make it clearer to anyone with a general interest, but without a scientific background.

When we deprive our body of food for longer than normal, for example during a fast, we notice changes in some of our hormones. As the levels of certain hormones change, this has a knock-on effect on different types of cells within our body. One of these hormones, Insulin-like Growth Factor 1 (IGF-1), is proven to decrease as we fast. IGF-1 is produced in the liver and is similar to insulin. Its purpose in the body is to make cells grow and produce new cells. When levels of IGF-1 decrease, our body produces fewer new cells and concentrates on repairing old ones. This state of 'repair' is very beneficial as it slows down the ageing process and may reduce the risks of cancer, diabetes and heart disease.

Another hormone that fasting seems to affect is a nerve cell growth factor in the brain, which changes the way neurons in the brain grow. This research is in its infancy and has yet to be tested on humans, but there are several indicators that suggest this is the mechanism that ultimately leads to a reduction in risk factors for cognitive diseases such as Alzheimer's.

There's a final exciting difference between standard calorie-restricted diets and intermittent fasting. Any weight you lose doing intermittent fasting is body fat! If this is not a reason to do the 5:2 diet over anything else then I don't know what is.

Other diets may show a decrease in body fat and muscle, but with intermittent fasting it seems to be just fat. Scientists are unsure at present why this is true, but it has been seen in a variety of studies so there is a good scientific basis for these findings. The most likely explanation is that when we fast, we have to use resources in our body (i.e. fat) for fuel rather than the food we have eaten. It may also be the key as to why the 5:2 diet is so successful for so many people.

Optimizing the benefits – do we need to skip meals?

The simple answer is yes. If your primary goal is health benefits, not weight loss, the science suggests you should eat only one meal on a fast day. Remember that how you consume calories over the fast day does not affect weight loss. Top scientists from the United States are in agreement that to get the absolute best out of intermittent fasting you need to either fast completely for 24 hours or, at most, have one small meal in the middle of the 24-hour period. The tests where they try other kinds of calorie restriction over the 24-hour period just haven't been done yet, so it's hard to tell for sure whether the science backs this up.

If you're reading this and thinking, Help, there's no way I can only eat once a day, then you're not alone. And this is why I do not advocate skipping meals **unless** it's something that appeals to you **and** it's something you can see yourself sticking to in the long term.

First and foremost this is because it does not affect the rate at which you slim. If your main objective is to lose weight **and** gain the health benefits that come with sustained weight loss, then stick to the 500/600 calories on your fast days, but do not worry about when you eat them.

Secondly, although the health benefits may not be optimized, you are still getting some of them. You are fasting and your body is going into repair mode so don't panic if you are not fully 'optimized'. Is anything in your life fully optimized? I know it's not the case for me.

Finally, and most importantly, what do you think is best: having a strict fast with only one meal but finding it so hard and de-motivating that you give up after a month **or** eating two or three small meals on your fast day and finding it sustainable in the long term?

I'd say the latter is by far the best option, but use your own preference. If you find it easier to skip a meal, then do so.

I often, but not always, skip lunch on a fast day. But if three meals a day works for you then don't change it. You are doing great as you are.

What's in a name?

There are many different names for diets that are the same or similar to the 5:2 diet, so it's no wonder people are getting confused.

The fast diet or 5:2 diet

These are, as far as anyone can tell, the same diet – just two names for the same thing. I think the double name comes from the origins of the diet. The 5:2 diet didn't exist before a TV programme by Michael Mosley in August 2012. Many people, including myself, started following the simple principle of eating less two days per week. At this stage it didn't have a name and as people were discussing it on Twitter and other social media sites it needed a name, so the simplest name stuck – the 5:2 diet. Later, as the diet became a phenomenon, marketing types got hold of it and it also became known as 'the fast diet'. In the US, where the diet never grew through word of mouth, it seems to be just called 'the fast diet' or 'the British fast diet'.

The 2-day diet

The 2-day diet has a totally different root to the 5:2 diet, despite its similarity in name and action.

The 2-day diet grew out of some amazing research by Dr Michele Harvie at the University of Manchester over the last few years. Harvie is a breast cancer specialist and has been looking at ways to reduce breast cancer risks through diet.

She has done experiments with groups of overweight women, where she radically changed their diets just two days a week. The diet has many similarities to 5:2, in that you restrict calories two days a week and eat normally for five. But the calories are restricted to 650 for both men and women and the food eaten on a fast day is more prescriptive – it includes a certain amount of milk and is totally carbohydrate free (rather like the Atkins diet) on the fast days. Most contrastive to the 5:2 diet is that the two days must be consecutive.

Her research highlighted two important things. First, that dieting two days a week was easier and that more people stuck to it than dieting all the time. Harvie compared two groups of women. The first group fasted two days a week and the second group followed a standard calorie-restricted diet, sticking to 1500 calories a day. After three months of following the diets, the research showed that intermittent fasters were almost twice as likely to stick to their diet.

The second and most impressive finding of her research was the reduction in a breast-cancer-causing hormone called leptin, which was reduced on average by 40 per cent, and a drop in insulin levels of 25 per cent, cutting the diabetes risk in these women.

Alternate day fasting (ADF)

Alternate day fasting originated in the US before the fast diet became popular in the UK. The principles of this diet are very simple. A strict fast diet is followed every other day. It also restricts how many meals you eat in that one day. The 5:2 diet is a variation on this theme, allowing you to fast for fewer days in a week and also to take weekends off. They are similar in terms of weight loss and effects, although obviously you may lose weight faster on ADF. But the success rate (i.e. the number of people who stick to the diet in the long term) is lower.

There has been an interesting study in the US by Dr Varady into ADF. Varady's research is fascinating. She took a group of both male and female overweight volunteers and started them on ADF for a year. This study is still progressing, but initial results in this case show a low dropout rate, gradual and continued weight loss and falls in both total and LDL ('bad') cholesterol.

Window or 8-hour fasting

Window fasting is a slightly different way of structuring your fast days. You fast for a part of your day, seven days a week. For example, a popular structure is that you fast from 8 p.m. on one day until 12 p.m. the following day. This means that your eating 'window' is 12 p.m. to 8 p.m. every day. Some people find that this kind of fasting fits more naturally into their lifestyle as they can eat a normal lunch and dinner every day, but it's definitely not to everyone's taste.

There has not been much research into this particular type of intermittent fasting, but the results are likely to be similar to that of 5:2 fasting or ADF.

Intermittent fasting (IF)

Intermittent fasting is a coverall term for any type of fasting diet. So the 5:2 diet, the fast diet, the 2-day diet and ADF all come under the umbrella of intermittent fasting.

The advantages of 5:2/fast diet over other forms of intermittent fasting

There is a reason why more people follow the 5:2 diet than any other form of IF – you are more likely to have success because it's easier to stick to and simpler to fit into your lifestyle. The dropout rate is lower than other types of IF and, indeed, than other types of diet. Put simply, the 5:2 diet is the simplest and most sustainable fast diet.

Possible dangers and side effects of the 5:2 diet

Because this diet is a fairly radical approach to weight loss, it is wise to speak to your doctor first to see if it is safe to follow the diet.

Current medical opinion suggests that the benefits of fasting are unproven. This is because long-term studies take several years, or even decades, to complete and this is a relatively new field.

The good news is that no significant dangers or problems with the diet have been reported so far. We can also take note that certain religions have been fasting for hundreds of years. Fasting during Ramadan requires Muslims to fast during daylight hours for a month. Fasting is also common among most Hindus. They fast on certain days of the week based on their belief and to appease certain deities. Both Hindus and Muslims believe that fasting is important for the wellbeing of human beings as it nourishes both physical and spiritual needs.

What about side effects?

As with all big changes to your normal diet and routine, there can be side effects. Some people will not experience any side effects, but a few will find the side effects to be so uncomfortable that they will be unable to continue with the diet.

Some of the side effects seem to occur only when fasting is first attempted. These effects, such as headaches and dizziness, will diminish and hopefully disappear altogether over a period of several weeks.

Dehydration seems to be a common side effect of following

the fasting diet that doesn't fade in time. It is easily dealt with by sipping plenty of water or other low-calorie drinks regularly throughout the fasting day.

What about irritability? Yes, some of us do get grumpy when we are feeling hungry. This does seem to reduce as we get used to fasting. But I can get grumpy on fast days and normal days too!

Some people report difficulties sleeping due to hunger and daytime sleepiness. This is less common than other symptoms. Most people feel a buzz of energy during their fasting days. Difficulties sleeping can occur, particularly if you eat the majority of your calories during the early part of the day. Increasing the size of the evening meal and making sure it is rich in complex, filling carbohydrates helps the body feel sustained until after we go to sleep.

Finally, here's one side effect that has affected me. I've been feeling the cold all through the winter, but particularly on fasting days. It has been a rather cold winter this year, but I have been suffering more than I would expect. The result has been an increased wearing of jumpers – perhaps two or three at a time and a higher heating bill. I take comfort in the fact that this is likely to mean that my body fat is reduced and the diet is working well.

Fasting and hypoglycaemia

If you suffer from, or might be suffering from, hypoglycaemia as a medical condition consult your doctor before beginning the diet.

The feeling of low blood sugar when you haven't eaten for a few hours is a common problem and one which I have suffered from in the past. It may put someone off fasting, because they feel that they need to eat every couple of hours to keep their blood sugar stable. The basic problem is that if you don't eat every three or four hours then you can become hypoglycaemic and therefore irritable, moody, light-headed and shaky.

This is an interesting phenomenon as only a small proportion of the population actually have a malfunction in their ability to regulate blood sugar levels. The rest of us, who do not have an underlying medical condition, do not have to worry about getting 'low blood sugar' while fasting. This is because the body is amazingly effective at regulating the sugar flowing around the blood.

A study in which young adults who have symptoms of hypoglycaemia went on a monitored 24-hour fast found that, while they reported 'feeling hypoglycaemic, their blood sugar levels remained normal. What to do if you are worried about having a 'blood sugar crash' during a fast period? This is a very real problem that I myself suffered from when I started the diet. I now know that my blood sugar levels are fine; I am in fact just exceptionally hungry. Here are my tips that helped me get through it, which I hope will help you too.

- Eat regularly during your fast day – this means three small meals.
- If you feel a wave of light-headedness coming over you, know that it will in all likelihood pass and you will feel normal again in 15 minutes.
- Finally, if it affects your ability to function normally or gives you a headache then you should eat something – nothing that big, ideally 100 calories or so of something filling, a slice of toast or a small banana, for example. Allow yourself those extra calories for that day, but carry on with the fast day if possible.

Don't let it put you off your next fast day, which will probably be easier. On your next fast day, see if you can last longer without feeling poorly.

When not to fast?

There are certain medical conditions that would make fasting inadvisable or even dangerous, even in this more restrained form. Don't attempt fasting if you are diabetic or pre-diabetic without seeking medical advice first. It is also not suitable if you are pregnant, breastfeeding or under 18 years old. If you are in any doubt, you must see your doctor first to discuss your options for dieting.

Those who are lucky enough to have good health and for whom fasting is a sensible diet option should also consider that there are some days that prove difficult for fasting.

If you're already a 5:2er, you will already know that some fast days will breeze by while others will be hard. There have been a few times where I have chosen not to fast or given up on a fasting day halfway through. I don't feel bad about this because I made the choice for the good of my short-term health and restarted the diet as soon as I felt better. Some of the things that have caused me to consider whether I should be fasting that day include a cold (it's hard to fast when you have a bad cold, so my advice is: don't fast), when I've had little or no sleep and possibly, for women only, at certain times of your monthly cycle.

Want to find out more about the health benefits?

Here are the studies referenced in this section. Be warned, most of it is not light reading, but it's a very exciting field and could be worth the effort. Finally, this list is not exhaustive. This is because research in this field is booming and there are new studies coming out all the time. Look out for breaking news stories, which I believe will show more proof and more reasons to fast.

1 Parrella E., et al. 'Protein restriction cycles reduce IGF-1 and phosphorylated Tau, and improve behavioral performance in an Alzheimer's disease mouse model', http://www.scribd.com/doc/126262180/Longo-Cohen-Paper.

2 Mattson M., et al. 'When a little poison is good for you', *New Scientist*, 6 August 2008, http://www.newscientist.com/article/mg19926681.700-when-a-little-poison-is-good-for-you.html.

3 Varady K., et al. 'Alternate day fasting (ADF) with a high-fat diet produces similar weight loss and cardio-protection as ADF with a low-fat diet Metabolism', pp137–143, January 2013.

4 Alken J., et al. 'Effect of fasting on young adults who have symptoms of hypoglycaemia in the absence of frequent meals', *European Journal of Clinical Nutrition* 2008; 62: 721–726.

THE MAGIC NUMBERS

How to customize the 5:2 diet for you

Everybody is different: different weight, different height and different fitness. In this chapter we work out your Body Mass Index (BMI) and metabolic rate (BMR), which is how many calories you burn in a day. By calculating your BMI, we can set suitable and sustainable weight-loss targets. By working out your personal metabolic rate we can set a personalized calorie intake guide for the fast days, and, as we know, every calorie counts on a fast day.

Recently, there have been improvements to the way the BMI is calculated. This is because the old scale of BMI didn't work very well if you were tall or short or more muscular than average; Brad Pitt, for example, at the time of *Fight Club* was very muscular and would have been considered overweight using the old BMI, so the new scale aims to be more accurate for everyone.

It doesn't make much difference if you are relatively average, but if you are short it can make your BMI higher and if you are tall it can reduce your BMI a little. If you are tall, like me, it's worth having a look at the new calculator – I dropped by 0.5 points from 21.6 to 21.1. But if you are average height it won't make a difference.

The simplest way to calculate your BMI is to use an online calculator, such as:

http://people.maths.ox.ac.uk/trefethen/bmi_calc.html

- A BMI of less than 18.5 is considered underweight.
- A BMI of 18.5 to 24.9 is considered a normal healthy weight.
- A BMI of 25 to 29.9 is considered overweight.
- A BMI of 30 or greater is considered obese.

Personalized calorie allowance on fast days

While we use the standard numbers of 500 calories as a quarter of a woman's normal daily calorie intake and 600 calories as a quarter of a man's, we can in fact be far more accurate.

By calculating your Metabolic Rate (MR) you can work out your daily calorie needs. The BMR is how many calories your body burns when at rest.

First calculate your BMR:

WOMEN

BMR = 655 + (4.35 × weight in pounds) + (4.7 × height in inches) − (4.7 × age in years)

For example my BMR is:
655 + (4.35 × 142) + (4.7 x 68) − (4.7 × 38) =
655 + 617.7 + 319.6 − 178.6 = 1414

655 + (4.35 × W)_____ + (4.7 × H) _____ − (4.7 × age) _____
= _____

Your BMR _____

MEN

BMR = 66 + (6.23 × weight in pounds) + (12.7 × height in inches) – (6.8 × age in years)

66 + (6.23 × W)_____ + (12.7 × H) _____ – (6.8 × age) _____ = _____

Your BMR _____

To calculate your actual calorie needs to maintain your current weight, you just need to work out where you are on the exercise scale.

Sedentary	Little or no exercise	BMR × 1.2
Lightly active	Light exercise Sports 1–3 days per week	BMR × 1.375
Moderately active	Moderate exercise Sports 3–5 days per week	BMR × 1.55
Very active	Hard exercise Sports 6–7 days per week	BMR × 1.725
Extra active	Very hard exercise Sports 7 days + physical job	BMR × 1.9

To work out the actual number of calories your body needs to maintain weight, multiply your BMR by the factor in the table above.

My maintenance calorie needs are:

I decide I am lightly active, so my multiplying factor is 1.375.
1414 × 1.375 = 1944 calories

I can also calculate how many calories I need to take in on my fasting days, as it is a quarter of this figure.

1944 ÷ 4 = 486 calories

So when I work out how many calories I am going to eat on a fast day, I need to make sure it is less than 486.

Your activity level _____

Your multiplying factor _____

(BMR) _____ × (MF) _____ = _____

Calories your body needs to maintain weight _____

Calories to eat on a fast day (÷ 4) _____

You should end up with the number of calories you need to eat on your fasting days. If you are like me, it will be slightly lower than 500 calories, but you might find you have a bonus of a few extra calories instead!

Don't forget, if you lose a lot of weight, but find it slackens off after a while, you might need to re-calculate your calorie intake, as these formulas depend on your weight.

There is also one more thing that is worth considering: there are about 3,500 calories in 1lb of stored body fat. That means you need to reduce your calorie intake by 3,500 to lose 1lb in weight. That might sound like quite a lot, but if you think of it in terms of the restricted calorie days, a woman has a calorie deficit of (2,000–500) = 1,500 per day on a fast day, so will reduce her calorie intake by 3,000 over a standard 5:2 week. For a man this figure is increased to a 3,800 calorie reduction. This means that without doing anything else, a woman will lose just under 1lb a week on the 5:2 diet; a man, just over 1lb.

Taking into account the level of exercise and healthy eating on non-fast days, then we are looking at an even greater weight loss. This is simple maths and doesn't take into consideration the effects that the 5:2 diet has on the body, which research is showing is more effective than standard diets.

GETTING STARTED

Now you know the basics it's time to get started and think about your first fast day.

Are you fit and well and ready to lose some weight?

The first thing to think about is what days would be most suitable for a fast. Remember, you need two days a week with at least one rest day in between. You can have a set routine and pick the same days every week or pick and choose. The diet is extremely flexible and is designed to fit in around you and not the other way round.

What days do you normally fast?

'Tuesdays and Thursdays. My husband is out so I don't have to worry about catering for anyone else on those days.'

Peggy

Monday is a common day to start as most people want to enjoy their food at the weekend and are ready to start the new week with good resolutions.

'I like to fast on a Monday, to get rid of that weekend bloat, and on a Thursday, in preparation for the weekend bloat!'

Jodie

Take a look at your schedule for the week and rule out any days where you have social engagements, especially involving food.

> 'My fast days are variable, depending on what I am doing that week. It changes from week to week.'
>
> **Christina**

Look at this as the greatest asset of the diet. Imagine going out for dinner with friends, not worrying about what you eat and even having a dessert and wine, and all the time losing weight.

Do the planning, do the fast days and then for five days a week, don't diet. Especially when you are first starting out, your diet days should be the least social days on your calendar. They are also likely to be busy days or work days, as you want to be distracted from food and away from the kitchen as much as possible. The only restriction on your fast days is that you must have a rest day between fasts.

Your first fast day will probably be the hardest as your body needs time to adjust to the new regime. So make sure you pick your days wisely when you start out. For the first two weeks you need to give careful consideration to when you fast as there is a possibility that you will feel lightheaded, grumpy and perhaps get a headache as well as feel properly hungry. Don't worry or be alarmed. There are plenty of tips here to deal with all these things. After the first two weeks of fast days, you will see it getting considerably easier. Focus on the fact that it's only one day.

Setting targets

Before you start you need to take your starting weight. Don't think about it too much – everyone's starting weight is high, otherwise you wouldn't be thinking about your diet. Think positively. Think how good you will feel when you start losing weight.

Starting weight:_____ st _____ lb

A few tips about weighing yourself

Don't worry about only weighing yourself once a week. You should weigh yourself when you like, just try not to do it every day as your weight can go up as well as down. We only care about the downward trend.

Ladies, be aware that your bodily cycle will have an impact on your weight. You may put on weight the week before your period and may also find fasting harder during this time. Try and stick with it and make allowances for your cycle if you find you haven't lost as much weight as you would like.

I would recommend weighing yourself the morning after your second fast day of the week. If you fast on Mondays and Wednesdays, then Thursday morning before breakfast or a drink and after you have been to the toilet is when you will be at your lightest. If you can, use this as your weekly weigh-in to see if you have lost weight and hit your target.

How much weight should you aim to lose?

This will depend entirely on your starting weight and fitness. If you have got more to lose, you will lose weight faster and can set a higher target. If you are quite close to your target weight and already reasonably fit, you won't be quite as quick but you will still lose weight.

The target for your weight loss should be between 1 and 4lb per week. This is not a crash diet and you should only be aiming to lose weight in a safe and sensible way.

As a general guide, if you are just fasting but not exercising you should aim to lose 1lb per week. If you are fasting, exercising and staying healthy on your normal days then you could potentially see a weight loss of 2–3lb per week.

If you have more weight to lose then your target could be potentially higher than that.

Target weight loss per week: _____ lb

	Weight	Weight lost	Target achieved?
Starting weight			
After 1 week			
After 2 weeks			
After 3 weeks			
After 4 weeks			

It is also worth calculating your BMI at the start and end of the four-week period. You should have dropped at least a couple of points and may even have crossed into a healthier bracket.

Starting BMI: _____
(Look in the 'Magic numbers' chapter on page 17 if you want help calculating your BMI.)

BMI at the end of the 4-week plan: _____

Looking at your body tone and fitness

Try looking at yourself in the mirror before you start, as it will help you see which areas you would like to look better for the summer. If you want to see the improvements, you need to see what you look like before as well, so ladies, put on your bikini or swimsuit, and gentlemen get your board shorts out. It's time to try them on and have a good look at yourself in a full-length mirror.

First of all, ignore the fact that you are probably a little pasty – everyone looks like that at the beginning of summer and we all know how to fix it. That is a different problem.

What you want to be looking at is where you think your problem areas are. Is it your tummy? Thighs? Cellulite? Or a little bit of everything?

The 5:2 Bikini Diet exercise programme is designed to burn as much body fat as possible while improving muscle tone, giving you a leaner, healthier body in just 30 days. Remember that the diet will help shift the excess pounds, specifically some of the fat. Where we need to help out with exercise is to bring some definition to the flab.

Exercising three times a week for four weeks, as well as following the 5:2 diet, will bring noticeable changes to your body shape. After four weeks put on your swimsuit again and see if you can spot the changes. Then slap on a bit of fake tan if necessary and get yourself to the beach!

Your first fast day

You need to do a bit of planning before you start on the first fast day. There are many different ways in which you can eat your 500/600 calories, but I would recommend that on your first day you have three small meals.

For women this means something similar to:
100 cals for breakfast, 150 cals for lunch, 250 cals for dinner

For men this could look like:
100 cals for breakfast, 200 cals for lunch, 300 cals for dinner

You should plan out exactly what you are going to eat. Take a look at the recipe section (see pages 77–210) for some inspiration. Try not to eat much carbohydrate as this is very calorific. Stick to lean meats, vegetables and complex carbohydrates such as pulses or beans. Don't consume too many calories in drinks. Drink black coffee or tea, diet colas, etc. An omelette (one large egg has 89 calories) makes a good, filling and simple meal. A salad is also a good option for lunch or dinner.

If you normally drink caffeinated drinks, don't cut them out, as a sudden lack of caffeine could give you a headache and make the fasting day harder. If you like milk in your tea or coffee just remember to count the calories. A cup of tea or coffee with (50ml/scant ¼ cup) semi-skimmed (low-fat) milk has 25 calories, made with skimmed milk it has 19 calories. A short skinny latte from Starbucks has 67 calories and a tall skinny latte has 102 calories.

You may find the evening rather long and drawn out too. As you have hopefully had 250–300 calories for your dinner you actually won't feel as hungry as you did during the day. But if you are at home with some snacks in the cupboard then you may well need some will power. Top tips to get you through your first fast day evening: find something good on the television, have a hot drink and go to bed early!

Remember:

- Feeling hungry is a natural state.
- Have a calorie-free drink to satiate your hunger.
- The first fast day is the hardest.
- You only have to do it once.
- Tomorrow you can eat like a king.
- You are actively losing weight right now.
- Feel proud and revel in a real sense of achievement.

Your first normal day

Congratulations on making it through your first fast day! If you want, you can weigh yourself before you eat or drink anything. You may well have dropped 1lb in your first day. Now, normally I would be suggesting that you eat healthily and don't snack on the day after a fast, but I think the rules can go out of the window on the first day. So you can eat what you like. Even though you have most likely been looking forward to your breakfast for most of the day before, you may find you are not as hungry as you thought. Or you may find you are starving and can't stop eating. Don't worry about it. It's just your body adjusting and you can allow yourself some treats.

I remember on my first normal day I didn't feel as good as I was expecting. The big breakfast made me feel tired and lethargic and I found it hard to get motivated all day. I have heard similar tales from others when they were just starting out with the 5:2 diet. These feelings will change quite dramatically as you continue with the diet. Just as the fast days get easier, the normal days get more, well, 'normal' really.

FAST DAYS

I suggested that you should eat three small meals on your first fast day. As you continue with the diet, you will probably want to adjust this to suit your body's needs and your lifestyle. It is normally wise to leave at least 50 per cent of your calorie intake for the day until your evening meal, although you can eat this meal as early as you like, any time after 5 p.m. But how you split your breakfast and lunchtime calories is more interesting. You could skip breakfast, skip lunch or have a small meal at each.

Here are a few questions that might help you decide how best to manage your meals on a fast day.

- Do you get up early?
- Do you work in an office?
- Are you exposed to unhealthy food during the day?

If you answered yes to some or all of the above questions then it might be worth considering missing breakfast and having a slightly more substantial lunch. Why? Because eating at lunchtime will make it easier to avoid snacks during the day. If you are rushing out first thing, you should find it easier to miss breakfast.

- Are you busy during the day with little time to think about food?
- Do you feel cranky if you skip breakfast?
- Do you have a morning ritual which involves breakfast and coffee?

If you answered yes to some of the above questions then you should try having a bigger (200–300 calorie) breakfast and then going through until your evening meal. Why? If you are busy at work you will not notice lunchtime.

If you are still unsure, stick to three small meals and perhaps adjust a little when you discover your hungriest times of day.

Count your calories

This is, I admit, the boring bit of a fasting day. You have to count calories and you need to do it accurately, without leaving anything out. Don't allow yourself any snacks between meals (except low-calorie drinks), as a snack will just waste your calorie allowance.

Read the packet of anything you are planning to eat, as practically all packaging will list the calorie content, then use one of the recipes in this book, which has been accurately calorie counted for you. Or, make up your own recipes, counting the calories in each individual component, using the calorie reference at the back of this book (page 235).

You will find that you have a few favourite dishes that you come back to time and time again. It's often omelettes or eggs in some form, or a salad. You will be able to work out the calories once and know for next time.

Feeling hungry – it's a good thing

I'm going to be totally honest here: you will feel hungry on your fast days. It may be a new kind of hunger that you have never experienced before, but it's not a bad thing. It won't make you ill and your body adjusts to it very quickly. This is because hunger is a natural state for our bodies, which haven't fundamentally changed since the Stone Age. Hunger makes us energetic and efficient and we use our coping mechanisms to find solutions to the hunger. In the old days this would have meant hunting for food. When we feel hungry by choice, this means finding distraction mechanisms.

'I have a drink to deal with hunger pangs or nibble on a carrot stick.'

Sarah

You will notice two positive things on your fasting days that you won't believe until you try it. First of all, you will have more energy, not less. It's unbelievable I know, but the majority of people on the 5:2 diet feel great on their fast days. I tend to feel lively, very chatty and have a natural buzz – the same kind of buzz that I get when I exercise. This feeling may not appear on the first fast day, but give it a week or two and start enjoying the feeling.

> *'I've had more energy, so the house is cleaner. The windows have never been so clean!'*
>
> **Deek43**

The second thing that seems a bit crazy before you start is that hunger comes in waves and normally passes in a few minutes if you think about something else. I tend to feel a real wave of hunger mid-afternoon, a time when in the past I would tend to snack unhealthily, but I now head out for some fresh air and don't think about food, and the feeling goes away. I might not feel hungry for another couple of hours and then it's nearly dinnertime and I'm on the home straight.

Special mention to mums at teatime

Are you a mother of young children? Do you struggle on a fast day at teatime? Because I do. With a meagre breakfast and/or lunch, by teatime I am hungry, and then I have to prepare food such as pasta or chips (French fries), which I can't eat. It's just the temptation to pick up the odd chip that I find really hard to resist, because I could do it without even thinking about it.

So if you find yourself in a similar situation, you are not alone. I try and eat with the children or soon after. This helps, as I know my food is on its way. If there's ever a time to employ the best of your willpower, it is now. Remember there are many mothers out there sharing your pain.

My backup plan after a hard day: fish fingers and beans, then we can all eat together. Two fish fingers and a quarter of a 415g can reduced sugar and salt beans has 220 calories and is very filling.

Fast day evenings

Do you eat your evening meal and then find the evenings rather long and boring? Do you find yourself constantly wishing you could eat some chocolate or cake? Don't worry, this happens to the best of us. You are probably not that hungry, it's just a bad habit, which is worse because you are relaxing.

Here are some of the things I like to do to keep myself busy and keep my mind off food until bedtime.

Take up a hobby – anything will do, something you do at home or go out to, as long as there's no food or drink involved.

Watch a movie – go to the cinema or put a movie on the TV. A movie is longer than a TV programme and if you are enjoying it, you won't be thinking about food.

Go for a swim – exercise is generally not a great idea on a fast day, but some gentle swimming is very distracting and no one is eating at the poolside.

Have a hot drink – fruit tea has no calories. I like peppermint myself. Another option if you have allowed yourself the calories is a low-cal hot chocolate drink. Normally around 40 cals, these will stop that chocolate craving.

'I make myself a black tea or glass of water, ring a friend and try to take my mind off it. It's only really bad just before I go to bed as I'm relaxing and nothing distracts me, but it doesn't last and when I wake up the next day, I'm no more hungry than normal.'

Deek43

Different ways of managing your fast days

Everyone has slightly different ways of managing their fast days. You may find there's a right or wrong way for you. Or you may find it develops over time.

'After the first week, I realized I had to adapt the diet to suit my needs. I start with a minute quantity of bran flakes and semi-skimmed [low fat] milk. Any diet of mine just has to include a minimum of three cups of tea plus a low-cal chocolate drink at night. I have a mug of Bovril for lunch and calculate all this at about 200 calories. I then have a proper dinner in the evening.'

Peggy

'Routine is key to the running of our household. I have breakfast at 7.15 a.m., a piece of fruit mid-afternoon and a light evening meal at around 7 p.m.'

Deek43

'I drink lots of water and limit myself to one cup of tea and one black coffee during the day. I keep myself totally busy so I don't think about food. I eat one meal in the evening, normally salmon and vegetables.'

Lou Piac

'I eat lunch (200 cals) and tea (300 cals).'

Jo

*'Three meals – 150 cals for breakfast, 150 cals for lunch and
200 cals for dinner.'*

Sarah

There are also plenty of tips about how to deal with the dreaded
hunger pangs. The most frequent is simply, 'By dreaming of
tomorrow!' but there are some other ideas too.

*'To deal with hunger pangs I drink a lot more fluid and look
forward to my hot drinks as though they were food. I tend either
to be more active in the evening or go to bed a bit earlier.'*

Rachel

*'I drink more fluid, which helps with hunger pangs. I also try
to do something interesting in the evening. I might go to the
cinema or the theatre. In fine weather, I'll go in the garden or
out for a walk.'*

Christina

*'I use drinks and snacks like Diet Coke, herbal tea, zero-fat
yogurt and miso soups to take away the hunger pangs.'*

Mikep

NORMAL DAYS

So now to the five normal days in a week. If you have tried the 5:2 diet before you may have heard the term 'feast' day bandied around for the non-diet days. This is a term I have made sure not to use here.

Let me explain. If you have tried the 5:2 diet before and found you didn't lose much weight or you lost weight at the beginning and then it tailed off to nothing, then you are one of many. Lots of people who have problems losing weight on the 5:2 diet have the same problem. We are eating too much on our normal days and negating all the good work we are doing on our fast days.

Let's look at me for example. In November 2012 I had been following the 5:2 plan for three months and was very close to my target weight. My plan was to continue following the plan right up to Christmas week, hopefully reaching my target weight in time for Christmas, and then I'd allow myself a week off. But as Christmas approached, although still sticking to my fast days, I stopped losing weight and even gained a pound or two. At the time I couldn't understand it. But as I re-examined my goals after Christmas I realized how much I had been eating on my normal days. I would allow myself the mince pies or chocolates or fancy canapés because I could eat what I liked and enjoy it. In fact, I ate far more than I have done in previous years at Christmas because I felt I was justified in doing this, as I was still on a diet. But I'm sure, looking back, that I was eating far more than my recommended daily calories. No wonder the diet was no longer working for me.

The revelation that I had in the cold light of January is that you cannot go crazy, binge and eat rubbish for five days a week. It just cannot work. For sustained weight loss and a healthy, long life, you need to eat healthily on your non-fasting days too.

The difficult truth is that it took me until the end of February to get back to the weight I was the previous November. So if you are reading this because you are finding that the 5:2 diet isn't working for you, then take a look at your 'normal' days and re-assess. The more people I have talked to about problems with the diet, the more often I find that this is the cause of a de-motivating failure of the 5:2 diet.

Since my moment of revelation in January, I have found a simple and logical solution. Feast days become normal, healthy days and the 5:2 diet is a winning formula once again. Here I set out the rules or suggestions that can make your normal days work for you. Don't worry, I don't suggest cutting out all fun and treats, but as with all healthy eating it involves saving snacks and chocolate for an occasional treat, rather than making them your standard diet. Your formula for a successful 'normal' day is as follows:

- Eat three healthy, balanced meals a day.
- Have light, healthy snacks such as fruit or yogurt if you feel peckish between meals.
- Do **not** calorie count or reduce portion size; you are not on a diet.
- Do be aware of what you are eating. Is it necessary? Is it healthy?
- Do allow yourself the occasional treat.
- Cut back on processed food and ready meals.
- Prepare home-cooked food as often as possible – the recipes in this book are just as good on a normal day as a fast day.
- If you are still hungry after a meal, wait 20 minutes and see if you are still hungry.
- Do allow yourself a glass of wine or two, a tasty dessert or even a few squares of dark (semisweet) chocolate.

Foods to avoid:

- biscuits (cookies) and cakes
- pastries
- crisps (potato chips)
- non-diet fizzy drinks
- chocolate bars and sweets (candies)
- beer, lager and cider

Use the recipes in this book as a guide for healthy, balanced eating. Just add rice, pasta and bread as necessary, but avoid processed additions.

Three of your normal days should also be exercise days. Try and get yourself into a good routine so the exercise becomes an integral part of your normal days. If you like, you can split your normal days into three healthy days with exercise and two normal days where you can be a little bit more relaxed. This means you can effectively have the weekend off. But remember, don't go overboard and cancel out all the things you have achieved during the week.

My schedule looks something like this:

Monday	Fast day
Tuesday	Normal and exercise day
Wednesday	Fast day
Thursday	Normal and exercise day
Friday	Normal and exercise day
Saturday	Normal and relaxed day
Sunday	Normal and relaxed day

Tweaking the 5:2 diet for greater weight loss

If you are reading this without reading the section above about eating healthily on your normal days, then please have a look. It is by far the most likely reason that you are not achieving the desired weight loss. If, however, you think you are eating healthily on those days but would like to give yourself an extra push, then there are a number of additional options worth trying in the short term to help you reach your goals.

One of the things to try is extending the window. This means increasing the length of time you are fasting. A standard window might be from the last thing you eat the night before the fast until the time you eat breakfast the following morning. So if you start the fast on Sunday at 10 p.m. and fast until Tuesday morning at 8 a.m. then the total fasting time would be 34 hours. To extend the window to an optimum 36 hours, you could just make sure that you don't eat after 8 p.m. on Sunday.

If, on the other hand, you find the 36-hour window a bit too long then you could try a 24-hour fast. This means starting at either 2 p.m. or 8 p.m. after lunch or dinner respectively and fasting until 2 p.m. or 8 p.m. the next day. This is slightly easier as you are eating a normal meal on both days, never having a full-day fast. This is also a good option if you don't want to lose weight but want to gain some of the health benefits of the diet.

Another way to extend the diet is to add another day, making it a 4:3 diet. Try this if you want to lose some extra weight. The days should be non-consecutive, such as Monday, Wednesday and Friday.

Finally, try a mix between the two. This is a kind of two-and-a-half-day diet. Have two normal days of fasting, say Monday and Wednesday – these are 36-hour fasts as described above – then have one day 24-hour fast day, say from 6 p.m. on Thursday to 6 p.m. on Friday. This is something I do occasionally and means I still get my relaxed weekend.

GETTING BEACH FIT

The 5:2 diet will help you lose weight and look and feel healthier, but to look good all over we need to look at body tone. The good news is that exercising just three times a week together with the two fast days will dramatically improve how you look and feel. There's no magic cure, but fasting plus exercise should even improve the appearance of cellulite. Remember, all exercise should be done on your normal days, not on your fast days.

What to do if you are unfit or don't exercise?

Start slow, but if you want to look good for summer I recommend walking or swimming. I wouldn't recommend starting on the exercise programme in Part 4 without improving your general fitness first.

Walking is exceptionally good for you as a starting point for exercise. It's free and very simple to start. Walk with a friend or take some music to listen to. Plan your route before you start and time yourself. You should be aiming to walk for 20 minutes, three times a week in the first week, increasing to 30 minutes, three times a week from the second week onwards. Your speed should be brisk with intent so it's not a dawdle, but it's not a speed test either. You should find that you naturally walk a little bit further every time you go out.

Swimming is another good way to get started with exercise. Choose your favourite stroke and swim gently, don't push yourself – for 20 minutes in the first week, increasing to 30 minutes when you can. You could also try water walking, where you walk up and down through the swimming pool. The natural resistance of the water makes this a great exercise technique to try.

The Sculpt 30 exercise plan

If you exercise or have an active lifestyle then this programme is for you. Even if you don't exercise regularly but are not sedentary then you can find success with this programme. This means if you are running around after active children or walk/cycle to work every day then you are ready to step up and look stunning for summer.

The 4-week plan on page 211 has been especially designed to fit in with the 5:2 Bikini Diet and your life. By following the programme three times a week on your normal days, you will notice considerable changes in your body shape and tone.

The plan uses a combination of resistance training (for your muscles) and cardio exercises to raise your metabolism and burn body fat for up to 24 hours after each session. The exercises can be done at home with some basic equipment or at your local gym.

The plan is quick and fun, so you don't have to spend hours on the treadmill. The training plan comprises 12 training sessions over four weeks that get progressively more difficult. For best results, make the three sessions a week part of your routine and don't let anything interfere with them. Remember, it's all about balance. Fitting this routine into your schedule is the simplest way to achieve amazing results.

Busting cellulite the 5:2 way

The 5:2 Bikini Diet is a fantastic way to reduce cellulite. Cellulite is just a type of body fat, but it is a horrible lumpy body fat that's deposited in all the worst places: hips, thighs and bottom. What's worse is that it has a dimpled 'orange peel' appearance that can make us feel self-conscious, especially in a swimsuit. The good news is that the 5:2 Bkini Diet is ideal for reducing cellulite, because when you lose weight through fasting, all the weight that you lose is body fat, and that includes cellulite.

The distinctive ugly appearance of cellulite comes from the fibrous tissue that only occurs in certain parts of the body like bottoms and thighs. In these areas, the fibres tether the skin to the muscle below. The cellulite is where the body fat bulges through the skin. The fibrous tissues cannot expand as the fat layer increases so we get the dimpled texture that we hate so much. You can't do anything about the fibres connecting the skin to the muscle so the only way to reduce cellulite is to reduce fat in these areas and to increase the tone of the underlying muscles. By fasting two days a week to reduce the fat and exercising to increase the tone, you should see a marked reduction in cellulite.

'*Most surprisingly my cellulite seems to have melted. It used to be all over my bottom and on my thighs, but now there's just a little bit on my bottom and I'm confident that will go too. I didn't expect that kind of result at all, let alone so soon.*'

Emma

There is a known medical process by which the body deposits fat on the hips and thighs. If we reverse that process then the fat will be removed from these areas first. An excess of insulin is one of the triggers for depositing fat in these areas. Intermittent fasting has been proven to reduce insulin levels, so that is one reason why the 5:2 Bikini Diet has an impact on cellulite in particular. Another trigger is an increase in oestrogen caused by pregnancy, the pill or HRT. If you are on the pill or HRT you may notice an increase in your cellulite. Other factors are smoking, too much alcohol and not enough exercise. If we keep these factors to a minimum, fast two days a week and exercise to increase muscle tone, we are doing everything possible to reduce cellulite.

QUESTIONS AND ANSWERS

Can I drink alcoholic drinks?

On a 'normal' day, yes, alcoholic drinks are definitely allowed. Obviously beverages that are higher in calories – such as beer and lager – should be kept in moderation, but wine and spirits are relatively low calorie and can be indulged.

On a 'fast' day I would not recommend drinking alcohol. It is unlikely that you can fit it in easily within your reduced calorie intake. If you do drink on a fast day it may make you feel light-headed and ultimately lead to you breaking the fast on that day.

Should I exercise on a fast day?

I wouldn't recommend exercising on a fast day, because you may feel weak and it will increase your hunger. However, some people do enjoy exercise on a fast day and do not suffer from any side effects.

Feasting – why can't I eat what I like when I'm not on a fast day?

If you wish to eat what you like on a 'normal' or 'feast' day, you can. You will still get some if not all of the health benefits of the fast diet. The change from 'feast days' to 'normal and healthy days' came about because some people, myself included, tended to binge rather too much on our 'feast days' and found we did not lose any weight. If you want to lose weight, you should eat healthily on your 'normal' days.

Should I eat all my calories in one meal on a fast day to optimize the health benefits of the diet?

The jury is still out on this one. Some US scientists believe that you need to eat no calories or eat only one meal to get the most of the health benefits, but the research to back this up is inconclusive at present. There's more information on this subject in the 'Health benefits' chapter (see page 6).

What type of food should I eat on a fast day?

The food you eat should be the most filling possible for the least amount of calories. The best things to eat are therefore lean protein-rich foods such as chicken or fish, and good carbohydrates such as pulses or beans. Salads and vegetables tend to have the least calories and can provide a big plate of food for very little calories. Have a look at the recipes in this book if you are stuck for ideas.

Why am I not losing weight quick enough?

Are you counting every calorie on your fast days? Are you sticking to a healthy diet on your normal days? Perhaps your target is too high; 1–2lb a week is a brilliant result. If you are exercising, some of your fat turns to muscle, which is heavier than fat. Have a look in the mirror and see if you can see body improvements.

Should I eat ready meals?

Healthy home-cooked food is best – it doesn't have to be complicated. Any processed food is likely to contain additional salt and preservatives and will have lost some of its goodness during production.

What about eating out?

On a 'normal' day I think a tasty meal out in a restaurant is a well-deserved occasional treat. Don't go overboard, especially if you tend to eat out more than once a week. Be careful and choose healthy options if you are eating at a fast-food restaurant or takeaway.

What do I do if I break the fast day rules?

Don't panic! If you have gone a little over your calorie allowance – anything up to 200 calories over – you don't have to give up on that day. Just watch what you did wrong and try and do it differently on your next fast day. If you totally fall off the wagon, call it quits and think about what went wrong the next day. Don't beat yourself up, and give yourself a little time off. Don't give up.

What about Christmas or holidays?

I think you should let yourself off. You won't lose weight and you may even put a pound or two back on. But you know that to lose it you just have to look forward to getting back to your fast days after your break. Bear in mind that it is likely that health benefits will decrease quickly when you take a break, but they will pick up where you left off when you start again.

I'm finding today's fast much harder than normal. Should I break the fast?

The first thing to try is to see if it passes. Is it a wave of hunger? I would wait for 20 minutes and see. If possible, get some fresh air. If that doesn't help then yes, I would break the fast. Your short-term health in this instance should take priority. It might be that you are coming down with something or, if you are a woman, it may be related to your cycle. Unless you recover very quickly when you eat normally again, I would suggest having a 'normal' day the following day as well and only do your next fast when you are feeling 100 per cent again.

NOT JUST A DIET, A WAY OF LIFE
Why everyone is raving about the 5:2 diet

For so many people with whom I have talked, the 5:2 diet has changed their life. It's not just about the slimming; it's a new healthier attitude to life. In short, it's inspiring.

Incredible, sustainable weight loss

'I have been steadily losing a pound a week since starting – only 2lb to go.'

Mikep

'I have been doing the diet for 10 weeks now and have lost 17lb. I'm 30 per cent of the way to my target weight. I'm confident I can reach my target weight, but know that this could take until the end of 2013.'

Lou Piac

'I've lost 8lb in one month so far. My target originally was to
get down to 10st (140lb), which would have been 7lb, but now I
have got the hunger for it (excuse the pun!) and have decided to
go for the whole stone (14lb)!'

Jodie

'I had been following a low-fat diet for some time but could not
lose the extra half stone (7lb) that I wanted to. Nothing worked.
But since starting 5:2 I have lost 6lb – only one more to go. I am
now at a weight that I haven't been for several years.'

Christina

'I lost an awesome 38lb in 3 months. The eating plan really
suited me and combined with my regular exercise and a sensible
balanced diet on the other days, the weight just dropped off.
I have been maintaining my target weight of 9st (126lb) ever
since, easily and happily. Still 5:2ing, but upping my non-fast
day cals to ensure that I maintain my weight.'

Lizzi

Why the 5:2 diet?

What makes the 5:2 diet so special and why do so many people
find the 5:2 diet successful? The majority of people have tried
other ways of dieting over the years. Some have had success but
have then found the calories creeping back up.

'I cut out all carbohydrates for three months. Horrid, but
effective. I couldn't sustain it and the weight piled back on
when I stopped.'

Peggy

'I have tried most diets over the last 25 years. Cambridge,
Cabbage, Weight Watchers, Slimming World, Rosemary Conley,
Atkins, Paul McKenna. You name it, I've tried it. All except the
baby food diet and a gastric band!'

Rachel

'I have tried calorie counting before and found it very difficult
to maintain the discipline of calorie counting every single day.
The degree of motivation and willpower required is difficult to
maintain. I am finding the 5:2 easier, because you only have to be
well-motivated two days a week and if you don't feel like it that
day, you just switch to another day.'

Mikep

Again and again I find people enthusing about the freedom that
dieting two days a week gives them. A lot of people find that
willpower and motivation is a lot easier to achieve over a single
day. There isn't the feeling of glumness that comes with so many
diets when you can't see a break. Is this the key to the success
of the diet?

'I like it because it doesn't involve permanent deprivation and
calorie counting. I find counting calories every day utterly soul-
destroying and I cannot sustain it for more than a few days. I'm
an all-or-nothing kind of person.'

Emma

'I like the fact that it is actually easier than you think to stick
to the fasting days and I like not feeling guilty about eating
normally on non-fasting days. I also like being more conscious
of the calorie content of things and think it makes me choose
healthy options on non-fasting days.'

Amy

'Thank goodness for the 5:2 diet. I love not having to work out
points or count calories for five out of seven days and not having
to worry if you are going out for dinner, etc. The 5:2 diet is so easy.'

Jodie

'I love that the 5:2 diet requires total discipline for only two days
out of seven. I find that I can manage this, and I know that I
have a feast day then to look forward to after each fast day.
In reality I find that I eat what I like and enjoy on the feast days,
but I do not indulge myself overmuch as my focus remains on
the ultimate goal. Not having to say to friends "So sorry, I am
unable to eat that because I am on a diet" is a total joy and
ensures that I never have to be either a pain for my hosts or
discourteous to them. If we are entertaining at home, we choose
one of my "feast days" for the occasion. Yes, the 5:2 does have
distinct advantages for me over other diets, and I love it.'

Lou Piac

For some people, the 5:2 diet has had an even more radical effect
on their lives and changed their attitude to food for the better.
This exceptionally positive outcome from Rachel has really
struck a chord with me.

'The most noticeable advantage for me is it has taken away all
the negative associations I have carried around with me about
food and eating over the last 25 years. I am enjoying food on my
normal days without feeling guilty. I've broken the pattern of
ridiculously over-eating, feeling guilty, beating myself up about
how greedy I am, leading to more over-eating. I'm feeling very
optimistic that the 5:2 is a way of life that is easy to stick to.
It allows me to really enjoy food that I like without feeling
guilty. I even look forward to fast days, and I find them very
manageable during a normal week.'

Rachel

What are the side effects?

There are some common side effects, but they don't seem to be putting anyone off the diet. To spare their blushes, I have not named people here.

- Lack of fibre has caused the odd digestive problem.
- Headaches and peeing.
- I do tend to fall off the wagon in the week of my period.
- Headaches on fast days for the first few weeks, but they have stopped now.

What do you eat on normal days?

'I eat in a normal healthy fashion. I treat myself to the occasional cake or pudding.'

Christina

'I eat sensibly on normal days, but I do enjoy a bit of chocolate or the odd glass of wine. But if I overdo it, I don't lose as much weight.'

Deek43

'I definitely don't eat more than normal. I think you get into a fasting mentality and I definitely check calorie content more and choose a healthier option. I also think it helps because if I do go out for dinner or have something "naughty", I don't feel too guilty about it – but I think I am still having those "treats" a lot less.'

Amy

'I eat less than I used to, weirdly, on my feast days. I think my stomach has shrunk and I am less hungry overall.'

Emma

What about exercise and body shape?

There's no right answer for how best to exercise, as this eclectic mix shows.

'I walk the dog three times a day, just over an hour in total every day. More at weekends.'

Deek43

'I exercise as part of life. I cycle with my kids in a trailer instead of using the car, walk several miles a day, swim once a week and try and fit in a yoga session.'

Jaime Fagan

'I have a treadmill and I use it every day. The diet and the exercise started simultaneously. My exercise routine had to start very gently; overdoing it simply stopped me in my tracks. By building up the speed and the time on the treadmill very gently, I have reached 22 minutes a day. As my weight falls and my fitness improves, I shall move up a gear on the treadmill, but for the moment both I and my GP are thrilled with the progress I am making.'

Lou Piac

'I do yoga three times per week. I walk a lot since my coaching practice involves taking people for beach walks. I feel a lot fitter.'

Lizzi

'I play golf, go to exercise classes and walk a lot. I have recently started t'ai chi.'

Christina

There have been some changes in body shape and image too. The most noticeable have been among people who have dieted and exercised. But those who haven't changed their exercise routine have benefited also.

'I've only been doing the diet for a month and have been unable to do any exercise due to major surgery on my feet. Amazingly I've noticed that my thighs are thinner and my tummy flatter.'

Emma

'I've got two children and my stomach is starting to take on its pre-childbirth appearance of relative flatness, instead of being convex. My bum appears to be more pert and my thighs are slimmer.'

Jaime Fagan

'Some small changes – particularly fitting into clothes better and my waist looking slightly thinner. Other differences have been having more energy and feeling more awake. It's hard to explain but my eyes feel more alert and open.'

Rachel

'I have dropped a dress size and have lost 2 inches from my waist, bust and hips.'

Hayley

How do friends and family respond to the diet?

Everyone seems to have very supportive family and friends, with plenty of them joining in once they have wised up to the health benefits.

'Everyone's just accepted my new routine. It's not impacted on their life, apart from not eating my kids' leftovers on diet days!'

Rachel

'Interested, and I have recruited a few friends too.'

Jo

'All very positive. My husband is even doing a version of it.'

Jaime Fagan

'Positively. My husband has accepted it and is pleased as he gets to eat lots of salad on fast days! He's not on the diet, but always thought I made portions too big. Friends are intrigued and want to know more, especially now they can see the results.'

Emma

'Accommodating, in awe and joining in!'

Lizzi

And what about the future?

Most people see themselves carrying on with the 5:2 diet into the future. In fact, some have already reached their target weight and have switched to a maintenance version. The important thing is that the 5:2 diet is viewed differently to every other diet. Everyone sees it as a positive life change, which they plan to continue in the long term.

'I would like to do it until I get down to my target weight and then I think I will go down to one fast day per week. Although if the weight starts to creep back on, I would go back to two days.'

Amy

'Actually, I see this being in my future. I think it is a healthy way of eating that's easy to maintain. It isn't sending a bad message to my daughter.'

Emma

'Forever is rather like never, one should not say either, simply because one never knows what the future holds. However, it is certainly my intention to keep to the 5:2 and to work within the flexibility it offers for the rest of the year, and most probably indefinitely.'

Lou Piac

'I think once I reach my target weight I will continue to use the 5:2 diet perhaps one day a week. This is to make sure my weight does not drift up again and, even more importantly, so that I continue to get the health benefits of the diet as I age.'

Mikep

'To me, it is so easy! Yes, I may be hungry for two out of seven days, but I can honestly say I look forward to that "empty" feeling on my fast days now and feel like it gives my body a rest. I am confident that this is for the long haul!'

Jodie

PART 2

THE

4-WEEK

PLAN

The 4-week plan is a detailed diet and exercise guide, which will give you the greatest weight loss and body definition. Here we take what has been learnt in Part 1: The 5:2 Bikini Diet and put it to good use.

If you follow this plan then you could lose up to 14lb in one month. You can achieve maximum weight loss if you are overweight with a BMI of over 25. You can find out your BMI in the 'Magic numbers' chapter (see page 17). If you are a healthy weight, with a BMI of between 18.5 and 24.9, then this plan is still perfect for you. Don't be disappointed if your weekly weight loss is slightly less.

This plan is also for you if you are lightly active or moderately active, i.e. you exercise between one and five times a week. It is also suitable if you don't exercise formally but are active in your daily life, by walking the dog, chasing after children or cycling to work.

If your lifestyle is currently sedentary but you are planning to exercise as part of the 4-week plan then use the exercise suggestions in the chapter 'Getting beach fit' (see page 40).

For each week there are targets to achieve; top tips; a suggested exercise schedule; what to expect that week and detailed menu plans.

Are you ready to lose weight, get slimmer and feel the healthiest you've ever been?

Remember the three golden rules for the 5:2 Bikini Diet:

1 Fast twice a week.
Two days a week you follow a calorie-restricted diet, that's:
- 500 calories for women
- 600 calories for men

The days are non-consecutive.

2 Eat normally but healthily on the other five days.

These are days when you are not on a diet. You should eat three healthy meals a day with limited snacks and treats in between.

3 Exercise three times a week on non-fasting days.

Follow the Sculpt 30 plan. You should try to increase the level of exercise or extend the length of time each week.

Now you know the simple rules you are ready to get started with Week 1 and your first fast day.

WEEK 1

Target weight loss: from 2–4lb

The changes in your body will be greatest in the first week. Try and enjoy the hungry feeling on your fast days and relish your food on the normal days.

Fast days

Start the week on a fast day. If you have never fasted before, try to eat three small meals. There are menu plans for both men and women with a plan for three small meals, a plan for breakfast and dinner, and a plan for lunch and dinner. Remember you can always swap menu plans as you discover what suits your body and lifestyle best.

Your first week of fast days is likely to be the hardest. You will need to be strict about counting calories and you are going to feel hungry. Think positively and just remember: you will find next week much easier.

Top tip! Drink plenty of water and low-calorie hot drinks. You may well be thirstier than normal and the drink will satiate your hunger pangs.

Normal days

To get the most from the 4-week plan, you need to be quite strict with yourself on your normal days too. Eat healthily, eat three balanced meals and cut back on unhealthy snacks.

Allow yourself a maximum of two treats during the first week on your normal days. A treat is a glass of wine, a dessert or some chocolate.

Exercise

Exercise three times over your normal days for 30 minutes each time. Follow the Sculpt 30 plan for Week 1 (see page 217–18. Don't forget to warm up beforehand and stretch afterwards.

Benefits that you are likely to see in the first week

If you have made it through the first two days of fasting, then you should be ready to congratulate yourself. The next week's fasting will be so much easier. Benefits such as increased energy are coming soon, but the first thing you will notice will be weight loss. Enjoy it!

Weigh yourself first thing in the morning the day after your second fast day. If you fast on Monday and Thursday, you should weigh yourself when you get up on Friday morning, before you eat or drink anything, but after you have been to the toilet. This is your weigh-in for the week.

Have you reached your target? Don't forget that you have still got your normal days to go. If you are on track, don't blow it by over-eating on your normal days. If you are behind target, be careful with your food on your normal days and weigh yourself again at the end of the week.

MENU PLANS FOR FAST DAYS: WOMEN (WEEK 1)

WOMEN: 3 SMALL MEALS

	Breakfast	Lunch	Dinner	Cals
Day 1	Egg white omelette with cherry tomatoes 84 cals (see page 80)	Basic salad with fat-free dressing 1 apple (53 cals) 132 cals (see page 94 and 96)	Harissa roasted chicken, shallots and sweet potato 261 cals (see page 161)	477
Day 2	Very berry jelly 1 satsuma (36 cals) 57 cals (see page 79)	Fragrant chicken broth 122 cals (see page 103)	Salmon with lemon mustard sauce 299 cals (see page 177)	478

WOMEN: BREAKFAST AND DINNER

	Breakfast	Dinner	Cals
Day 1	Mushroom frittata 265 cals (see page 151)	Chicken with ginger and mango sauce 234 cals (see page 138)	499
Day 2	Raisin and cranberry porridge 215 cals (see page 90)	Spicy prawn stir-fry 289 cals (see page 182)	504

WOMEN: LUNCH AND DINNER

	Lunch	Dinner	Cals
Day 1	Mozzarella and tomato salad 166 cals (see page 105)	Caribbean-style pork 299 cals (see page 170)	465
Day 2	Roasted red pepper couscous 216 cals (see page 119)	Spicy prawn stir-fry 289 cals (see page 182)	505

MENU PLANS FOR FAST DAYS: MEN (WEEK 1)

MEN: 3 SMALL MEALS

	Breakfast	Lunch	Dinner	Cals
Day 1	Egg white omelette with cherry tomatoes 84 cals (see page 80)	Halloumi salad 1 apple (53 cals) 268 cals (see page 117)	Harissa roasted chicken, shallots and sweet potato 261 cals (see page 161)	613
Day 2	Frozen berry smoothie 153 cals (see page 88)	Fragrant chicken broth 122 cals (see page 103)	Salmon with lemon mustard sauce 299 cals (see page 177)	574

MEN: BREAKFAST AND DINNER

	Breakfast	Dinner	Cals
Day 1	Raisin and cranberry porridge 1 satsuma *(36 cals)* *251 cals* (see page 40)	Simple jerk chicken with 40g (1½oz) basmati rice *(141 cals)* *352 cals* (see page 137)	**603**
Day 2	Mushroom frittata *265 cals* (see page 151)	Pork and apricot skewers with basic salad *286 cals* (see page 169 and 94)	**551**

MEN: LUNCH AND DINNER

	Lunch	Dinner	Cals
Day 1	Mozzarella and tomato salad 1 apple *(53 cals)* *219 cals* (see page 105)	Simple jerk chicken with 40g (1½oz) basmati rice *(141 cals)* *352 cals* (see page 137)	**571**
Day 2	Roasted red pepper couscous *216 cals* (see page 119)	Baked salmon on asparagus Raspberry cream *379 cals* (see pages 178 and 203)	**595**

WEEK 2

Target weight loss: from 2–4lb

Your body is just starting to adjust to the diet now. You will notice the fast days will be a little bit easier and your clothes may be looser.

Fast days

Again, try to start the week with a fast day. Week 2 is all about building on Week 1 and getting your body used to fasting. You should find the hunger pangs are milder and less frequent.

Top tip! If you feel hungry mid-afternoon (a common time for hunger pangs), distract yourself by going for a walk. The wave of hunger will soon pass.

Normal days

Stay healthy and don't over-indulge. You are allowed a maximum of three treats over the week on normal days.

Exercise

Follow the Sculpt 30 exercise plan for Week 2 (see pages 219–20). The exercises get progressively harder to maximize results.

At the end of the week

Have you reached your target weight? If you weigh yourself after the second fast day and you are not quite on target, stay healthy and make sure you exercise. Consider adding a third fast day in next week.

Do you feel healthier and more energized?

MENU PLANS FOR FAST DAYS:
WOMEN (WEEK 2)

WOMEN: 3 SMALL MEALS

	Breakfast	Lunch	Dinner	Cals
Day 1	Asparagus wrapped in Parma ham *99 cals* (see page 82)	Basic salad with fat-free dressing *79 cals* (see pages 94 and 96)	Grilled chicken topped with sun-dried tomatoes and olives *317 cals* (see page 160)	495
Day 2	Peppered egg *99 cals* (see page 81)	Mushroom stir-fry *146 cals* (see page 101)	Spanish fish stew *247 cals* (see pages 145–6)	492

WOMEN: BREAKFAST AND DINNER

	Breakfast	Dinner	Cals
Day 1	Pink porridge *151 cals* (see page 90)	Tuna and bean salad *306 cals* (see page 118)	457
Day 2	Overnight oats 1 satsuma *(36 cals)* *232 cals* (see page 89)	Mediterranean chicken with basil and feta *259 cals* (see pages 159–60)	491

WOMEN: LUNCH AND DINNER

	Lunch	Dinner	Cals
Day 1	Cajun roasted vegetables 175 *cals* (see page 109)	Tuna and bean salad 306 *cals* (see page 118)	**481**
Day 2	Flatbread (or mini naan) with feta and olives 289 *cals* (see pages 112–13 and page 115)	Mediterranean chicken with feta 259 *cals* (see pages 159–60)	**548**

MENU PLANS FOR FAST DAYS: MEN (WEEK 2)

MEN: 3 SMALL MEALS

	Breakfast	Lunch	Dinner	Cals
Day 1	1 egg on 1 medium slice granary toast 181 *cals*	Quick fried chickpeas with rocket 200 *cals* (see page 121)	Baked fish parcel 197 *cals* (see page 126)	**578**
Day 2	Strawberry smoothie 153 *cals* (see page 85)	Basic salad with Cheddar cheese 168 *cals* (see pages 94–5)	Butternut squash with rustic beans and chorizo 281 *cals* (see page 173)	**602**

MEN: BREAKFAST AND DINNER

	Breakfast	Dinner	Cals
Day 1	½ × 400g (14oz) can tomatoes on 1 thick slice granary toast 156 *cals*	Prawn green curry with 40g (1½oz) basmati rice (141 *cals*) 404 *cals* (see page 181)	560
Day 2	Overnight oats 196 *cals* (see page 89)	Salmon with lemon mustard sauce and 3 new potatoes (101 *cals*) 400 *cals* (see page 177)	596

MEN: LUNCH AND DINNER

	Lunch	Dinner	Cals
Day 1	Stuffed avocado 284 *cals* (see page 120)	Maple-glazed pork 295 *cals* (see page 168)	579
Day 2	Flatbread (or mini naan) with garlicky tomato sauce and anchovies 224 *cals* (see pages 112–13 and 115)	Sizzling pork boats with 40g (1½oz) basmati rice (141 *cals*) 371 *cals* (see page 143)	595

WEEK 3

Target weight loss: from 1–3lb
Your body is getting used to the diet now. This means that your weight loss may be slightly reduced. You are halfway through already!

Fast days

Your fast days should be getting a lot easier now, fitting in nicely with your routine. If you didn't hit your target weight loss in Week 2, you could add a third fast day this week.

Top tip! Allow yourself a low-cal chocolate drink in the evenings to quash those chocolate cravings.

Normal days

Stay strong on your normal days for the best slimming results. You are allowed up to four treats over the week. A treat could be a glass of wine, a dessert or some chocolate.

Exercise

You should now be on Week 3 of the Sculpt 30 programme (see page 221).

At the end of the week

Are you feeling great now? Energized by the diet and exercise? Slimming down fast? Your weight loss so far could be anything from 5lb to 12lb. You should also be able to see changes in your body shape. Only one week to go!

MENU PLANS FOR FAST DAYS: WOMEN (WEEK 3)

WOMEN: 3 SMALL MEALS

	Breakfast	Lunch	Dinner	Cals
Day 1	Low-fat plain or fruit yogurt 100 cals	Fresh garden soup 97 cals (see page 91)	Chilli beef stew with 30g (1¼ oz cup) basmati rice 310 cals (see page 141–2)	507
Day 2	Apricot, banana and cashew snack jar 99 cals (see page 83)	Basic salad with lemon vinaigrette 99 cals (see pages 94 and 96)	Simple jerk chicken with 2 new potatoes (68 cals) 279 cals (see page 137)	477

WOMEN: BREAKFAST AND DINNER

	Breakfast	Dinner	Cals
Day 1	Smoked salmon and cream cheese parcels 137 cals (see page 87)	Tuna and bean salad (see page 118) Pears poached in lemonade (see page 198) 372 cals	509
Day 2	Ham omelette made with 2 large eggs and 1 slice ham 219 cals	Pork and apricot skewers 286 cals (see page 169)	505

WOMEN: LUNCH AND DINNER

	Lunch	Dinner	Cals
Day 1	Roasted sweet potato with quick-cook chilli vegetables 181 cals (see page 110)	Coriander and lemon chicken with 3 new potatoes (101 cals) 300 cals (see page 123)	**481**
Day 2	Stuffed courgette rolls 121 cals (see page 102)	Chorizo and chickpea stew with 40g (1½oz) basmati rice (141 cals) 345 cals (see page 142)	**466**

MENU PLANS FOR FAST DAYS: MEN (WEEK 3)

MEN: 3 SMALL MEALS

	Breakfast	Lunch	Dinner	Cals
Day 1	Grilled portobello mushrooms 78 cals (see pages 81–2)	Basic salad with ham and honey mustard dressing 130 cals (see pages 94–5, 97)	Spicy prawn stir-fry with 50g (1½oz) noodles (100 cals) 389 cals (see page 182)	**597**
Day 2	Omelette made with 1 large egg 89 cals	Mozzarella and tomato salad 166 cals (see page 105)	Salmon baked with herbs Peach sorbet 334 cals (see page 196)	**589**

MEN: BREAKFAST AND DINNER

	Breakfast	Dinner	Cals
Day 1	Ham omelette made with 2 large eggs and 1 slice ham *219 cals*	Honey mustard chicken skewers with 4 new potatoes *(135 cals)* *335 cals* *(see page 124)*	554
Day 2	Smoked salmon and cream cheese parcels *137 cals* *(see page 87)*	Fresh tuna Niçoise with 2 large boiled eggs *(178 cals)* *446 cals* *(see page 150)*	583

MEN: LUNCH AND DINNER

	Lunch	Dinner	Cals
Day 1	Stuffed pepper with mushrooms and pine nuts *187 cals* *(see page 111)*	Quick turkey Bolognese with 50g (1¾oz) spaghetti *391 cals* *(see page 140)*	578
Day 2	Flatbread (or mini naan) with courgette and tomato 1 apple *(53 cals)* *269 cals* *(see pages 112–114)*	Baked fish parcel with 4 new potatoes *(135 cals)* *332 cals* *(see page 126)*	601

WEEK 4

Target weight loss: from 1–3lb
This is the last week of the plan. Are you on target? As this is your last week, do as much exercise as you can for maximum results.

Fast days

Keep on track during your fast days. Consider whether you can continue with one or two fast days per week after the plan is finished for sustained weight loss and health benefits.

Top tip! Plan a trip to the cinema or theatre for a fasting day treat. With something exciting to do, the evening will fly by.

Normal days

Carry on with the healthy eating. You are now allowed one treat a day, but don't get carried away!

Exercise

Complete the exercise programme for Week 4 (see pages 222–23). Make time for your exercise this week and push yourself in all of the exercises to the best of your ability. This will give you the best results.

MENU PLANS FOR FAST DAYS:
WOMEN (WEEK 4)

WOMEN: 3 SMALL MEALS

	Breakfast	Lunch	Dinner	Cals
Day 1	Melon with Parma ham 78 cals (see page 191)	Harissa olives 1 satsuma (36 cals) 128 cals (see page 187)	White fish with chilli and ginger sauce 40g (1½oz) basmati rice (141 cals) 281 cals (see page 127)	487
Day 2	Blackberry and almond snack jar 98 cals (see page 83)	Miso broth 117 cals (see page 100)	Stuffed avocado 284 cals (see page 120)	499

WOMEN: BREAKFAST AND DINNER

	Breakfast	Dinner	Cals
Day 1	Peppered egg 99 cals (see page 81)	Pork stir-fry with water chestnuts with 50g (1¾oz) noodles (100 cals) 389 cals (see page 166)	488
Day 2	Overnight oats 196 cals (see page 89)	Butternut squash with rustic beans and chorizo 281 cals (see page 173)	477

WOMEN: LUNCH AND DINNER

	Lunch	Dinner	Cals
Day 1	Homemade tortilla chips and salsa 1 apple (53 cals) 196 cals (see pages 192–3 and page 184)	Peppered beef with mustard sauce 296 cals (see pages 163–4)	492
Day 2	Basic salad with pastrami and honey mustard dressing 121 cals (see pages 94–5 and page 97)	Grilled chicken topped with sun-dried tomatoes and olives with 2 new potatoes (68 cals) 385 cals (see page 160)	506

MENU PLANS FOR FAST DAYS: MEN (WEEK 4)

MEN: 3 SMALL MEALS

	Breakfast	Lunch	Dinner	Cals
Day 1	1 large egg, scrambled, on 1 wholemeal (wholewheat) toast 189 cals	Roasted pak choi 98 cals (see pages 92–3)	Salmon and cucumber skewers 317 cals (see page 176)	604
Day 2	Pecan nut and fresh blueberry snack jar 99 cals (see page 83)	Basic salad with 20g (¾oz) chorizo 123 cals (see pages 94–5)	Roasted pork with plums and 3 new potatoes 374 cals (see page 167)	596

MEN: BREAKFAST AND DINNER

	Breakfast	Dinner	Cals
Day 1	Mushroom frittata 265 *cals* (see page 151)	Chicken satay with 30g (1¼oz) basmati rice (106 *cals*) 350 *cals* (see page 135)	**615**
Day 2	¼ × 400g (14oz) can reduced sugar beans on 1 thick slice toast 173 *cals*	Peppered beef with mustard sauce and 4 new potatoes (135 *cals*) 431 *cals* (see pages 163–4)	**604**

MEN: LUNCH AND DINNER

	Lunch	Dinner	Cals
Day 1	Chilli chicken salad 1 apple (53 *cals*) 324 *cals* (see pages 158–9)	Baked salmon on asparagus 271 *cals* (see page 178)	**595**
Day 2	Roasted red pepper couscous 216 *cals* (see page 119)	Sweet onion chicken with 40g (1½oz) basmati rice (135 *cals*) 370 *cals* (see page 139)	**586**

THE RESULTS

Congratulations! You have finished the plan. If you have followed the diet and done plenty of exercise I defy you to not feel better, look better and be significantly slimmer than you were just four weeks ago. If you haven't quite achieved enough weight loss, carry on with the 5:2 Bikini Diet for another couple of weeks to see if you can hit your goals.

Now is the time to take a look in the mirror and see if you look different. Are you slimmer? Areas where you may notice a difference are your tummy, bottom and thighs. If you have had problems with cellulite you might see that it's a lot less pronounced than before. Do you have a glow that you didn't have before? Have you had positive comments about your appearance?

The health-giving effects of the diet combined with exercise should energize you and make you perkier than ever before. Enjoy it! It's the new you. Get ready to hit the beach, the barbecue and the best summer parties. If you want to keep this feeling and this figure forever, read on to discover how to maintain your results into the future.

BEYOND THE 4-WEEK PLAN

If the 4-week plan has made for a new, slimmer and healthier you then there's more good news. It's really easy for you to continue with a few key points of the diet to maintain your weight and the health benefits in the long term.

Sustaining the diet

Take your foot off the pedal. The aim of the 4-week plan was to achieve maximum weight loss in a short period of time. Now is the time to enjoy yourself a little bit more without short-circuiting all of your hard work. If you are at your target weight, then you should look at a maintenance version of the 5:2 Bikini Diet. The simplest way to do this is to swap to one fast day per week. This should maintain many of the health benefits and allow you to keep a stable weight.

If you have still got a bit more weight to lose then don't worry. The 5:2 Bikini Diet is a great plan to continue for the next six months or a year. Carry on with the two days fasting and five days of healthy eating and you can't go wrong.

If your weight plateaus, check what you are eating on your normal days and see if you are having a few too many calories. Cut back and be as healthy as possible every day.

What about exercise? Instead of following a strict exercise plan, you can now pick exercises that you enjoy to help you keep fit and full of energy. Don't stop! If you have enjoyed the results of the Sculpt 30 programme, you can find out more about their advanced online training programme on their website, **www.sculpt.me.uk.**

The 5:2 – not a diet, a way of life

For many of us the 5:2 diet is so much more than a diet; it is a way of life. By carrying on with this lifestyle you are keeping slim and giving yourself a great chance of future health and happiness. Have you learned to love fasting? Do you see it as something you can carry on into the future? Congratulations! You have joined the fast diet revolution!

PART 3

THE

RECIPES

The recipes selected here are low in fat, rich in protein and with a restrained amount of slow-burning carbohydrates.

Good carbohydrates are complex (low GI) carbohydrates that are used more slowly in the body. They keep you feeling fuller for longer. Examples of good carbohydrates are lentils, beans and whole grains.

High-quality and lean proteins such as fish, chicken, lean red meat and eggs are a vital part of many of the recipes. They also help to keep you feeling full.

Every single recipe is suitable for a fast day, with fewer than 300 calories per portion. Each individual ingredient is calorie counted so you can make your own adjustments with a minimum of fuss. Although a few recipes require a smaller portion size, most provide you with a healthy, 'normal' plate of food. But don't just use these recipes on your fast days – they are perfect for any day of the week; just right to put a spring in your step on normal days too. On a normal day you should feel free to add extra carbohydrate if you wish. Simply add a portion of rice, pasta or potato or a slice of bread.

Many of the recipes are for one – for when it's just you fasting. In particular, the recipes with very few calories are almost all a one-portion size. For main meals there is a mixture of meals for one, two and four. The meals for two are perfect for sharing with a partner – I doubt you will get any complaints about 'diet' recipes. Remember you can always keep the second portion for another day. The recipes for more people are either for feeding your family or guests, or can be frozen in portions to provide an easy and healthy 'ready meal'.

BREAKFAST

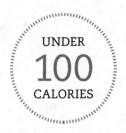

UNDER
100
CALORIES

Very berry jelly

21 calories

This is a refreshing fruity treat to start your fasting day off on the right track.

Serves 4   Preparation time: 5 minutes, plus 2 hours setting

1 × 23g (1oz) packet sugar-free raspberry jelly (32 cals)
....
100g (3½oz) fresh raspberries (25 cals)
....
100g (3½oz) fresh strawberries (27 cals)
....

- Make up the jelly according to the packet instructions BUT use 50ml (scant ¼ cup) less water than the instructions suggest. Divide the berries equally between 4 small glasses or ramekins, then pour the jelly over the fruit and leave in the fridge for about 2 hours or until set.

Egg white omelette with cherry tomatoes

84 calories

Egg whites are a good choice if you are cutting back on calories, as there are only 18 calories in an egg white.

Serves 1   Preparation time: 5 minutes   Cook time: 5 minutes

3 large eggs (54 cals for egg whites)
1 tbsp skimmed milk (5 cals)
3 sprays light sunflower oil (3 cals)
10 cherry tomatoes, cut in half (22 cals)
fresh basil leaves, torn (optional)
salt and freshly ground black pepper

- First, separate the eggs. Crack one of the eggs on the side of a clean bowl and, using your thumbs, open the two halves, letting some of the white run into the bowl. Carefully pass the egg yolk from one half of the shell to the other, letting the egg white run into the bowl. Keep passing the egg yolk from one half of the shell to the other without breaking it until all the white is in the bowl. Put the yolk in a separate bowl and repeat for the other 2 eggs. Add the milk to the egg whites and whisk together with a fork.
- Spray the oil into a wide frying pan (skillet) and warm over a medium heat for at least 2 minutes. Pour in the egg white mixture, then add the cherry tomatoes and basil immediately. Season with salt and pepper and cook until set. You may need to swirl and tilt the pan to distribute the eggs, tomatoes and basil evenly over the base of the pan. The omelette should cook in less than a minute. Serve straight away.

Peppered egg

99 calories

Serves 1   Preparation time: 2 minutes   Cook time: 6 minutes

¼ green (bell) pepper, diced (6 cals)
....
1 large free-range egg (89 cals)
....
2 tsp skimmed milk (4 cals)
....
salt and freshly ground black pepper
....

- Heat a small non-stick frying pan (skillet) over a medium heat. Add the diced pepper and dry-fry for 4 minutes until the pepper is tinged with brown.
- Meanwhile, crack the egg into a bowl, add the milk and whisk together with a fork. Pour the egg mixture into the frying pan and stir constantly until just cooked, but not runny. Season with salt and pepper and serve immediately.

Grilled portobello mushrooms

78 calories

Serves 1   Preparation time: 5 minutes   Cook time: 10 minutes

2 flat open or portobello mushrooms (32 cals)
....
1 tsp extra-virgin olive oil (27 cals)
....
½ garlic clove, peeled and crushed (2 cals)
....
1 tsp chopped fresh parsley
....
1 medium tomato (17 cals)
....
salt and freshly ground black pepper

continued

- Preheat the grill (broiler).
- Prepare the mushrooms by brushing off any soil and cutting out the stalks. Finely chop the stalks and mix in a small bowl with the olive oil, garlic and parsley.
- Cut the tomato in half, scoop out and discard all the seeds, then finely chop the tomato flesh and add to the bowl.
- Place the mushrooms open side down on a grill pan and grill (broil) for 4 minutes. Remove the mushrooms from the grill pan and turn them over. Distribute the garlic and tomato mixture evenly over the mushrooms, season with salt and pepper and grill for a further 6 minutes. Serve immediately.

Asparagus wrapped in Parma ham
99 calories

This will bring a little bit of class to your breakfast time, or indeed to any time of day.

Serves 1   Preparation time: 2 minutes   Cook time: 5 minutes

12 asparagus spears (45 cals)
2 slices Parma ham (prosciutto) (54 cals)
freshly ground black pepper
1 lemon wedge, to serve (optional)

- Cook the asparagus in a pan of simmering water for 4–5 minutes, depending on thickness.
- Cut the Parma ham (prosciutto) in half lengthways so you have 4 long strips. Remove the asparagus from the water and divide it into groups of three, then wrap the Parma ham around the stems. Arrange the wrapped asparagus piled up on a plate, season with pepper and serve with a lemon wedge on the side.

Breakfast snack jars

These little snack jars are a great way to have a healthy 100 calorie break-fast on the run. Find yourself a small lidded jar, such as an empty jam jar, and fill it with the ingredients in advance. These can even be prepared the night before. I have listed a few of my favourite combinations here, but there are an infinite number of variations, so please see the chart on page 84 showing the possible ingredients and their calories.

Serves 1   Preparation time: 2 minutes

Blackberry and almond snack jar

98 calories

6 whole almonds (73 cals)

20 blackberries (fresh or frozen) (25 cals)

Pecan nut and fresh blueberry snack jar

98 calories

2 pecan nuts (82 cals)

30g (1oz) fresh blueberries (18 cals)

Apricot, banana and cashew snack jar

99 calories

5 cashew nuts (57 cals)

2 dried apricots (16 cals)

1 tsp dried banana (26 cals)

Make your own snack jar

Use the chart below to work out how many calories are in your favourite combination.

1 almond	12 cals
10g (1/3oz) flaked (slivered) almonds (1 level dessertspoon)	61 cals
1 cashew nut	9 cals
1 pecan nut	41 cals
1 Brazil nut	20 cals
1 dried date	14 cals
25g (1oz) dried banana (1 rounded tbsp)	128 cals
1 dried apricot	8 cals
1 dried fig	45 cals
10g (1/3oz) dried pineapple (1 level dessertspoon)	28 cals
1 prune	21 cals
10g (1/3oz) raisins (1 level dessertspoon)	27 cals
1 ring dried apple	15 cals
10g (1/3oz) sunflower seeds (1 level dessertspoon)	58 cals
10g (1/3oz) pumpkin seeds (1 level dessertspoon)	57 cals
1 blackberry	1 cal
1 medium strawberry	3 cals
1 raspberry	1 cal
25g (1oz) fresh blueberries (1 rounded tbsp)	14 cals
1 tbsp dried cranberries	81 cals

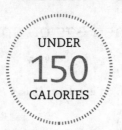

UNDER
150
CALORIES

Strawberry smoothie

147 calories

You can also make this with raspberries (about 20) for a raspberry smoothie, if you like.

Serves 1   Preparation time: 5 minutes

5 strawberries, hulled (20 cals)
½ banana (53 cals)
1 tbsp fat-free plain yogurt (10 cals)
200ml (generous ¾ cup) skimmed milk (64 cals)

- This is a simple one. Place all the ingredients in a blender and whizz until smooth. Serve immediately.

Poached egg on spinach

103 calories

I learned how to poach an egg from Delia's *How to Cook* and it has never failed me yet.

Serves 1　Preparation time: 5 minutes　Cook time: 12 minutes

1 large free-range egg (89 cals)

50g (1¾oz) fresh baby spinach leaves (12 cals)

juice of ½ lemon (2 cals)

salt and freshly ground black pepper

- Half fill a wide saucepan with water (it needs to be at least 2.5cm/1in deep). Heat the water until it is bubbling gently from the base of the pan, then carefully crack the egg on the side of the pan and lower gently into the water – you want to disturb the egg as little as possible at this point. Check that the water is still bubbling, but only just, then set a timer for exactly 1 minute. Take the pan off the heat and leave the egg in the hot water for another 10 minutes.
- Meanwhile, put the spinach, lemon juice and a little salt and pepper in a small pan and heat over a medium-high heat. Cover with a lid and cook for exactly 2 minutes. Transfer the spinach to a small serving plate, gently squeezing out any extra liquid from the spinach as you do so.
- Using a slotted spoon, carefully remove the egg from the water and place on top of the spinach. Eat immediately.

Smoked salmon and cream cheese parcels

137 calories

These parcels need a little preparation, but they can be made the night before and refrigerated.

Serves 1 (makes 2 parcels)   Preparation time: 10 minutes

2 tbsp light soft cheese (50 cals)
juice of ½ lemon (2 cals)
freshly ground black pepper
60g (2¼oz) smoked salmon, about 4 small slices (85 cals)
1 lemon or lime wedge, to serve

- In a small bowl, mix together the soft cheese, lemon juice and black pepper.
- Lay two pieces of salmon out in a cross shape, then place a large dollop of the cream cheese mixture in the middle of the cross. Bring up the sides of the salmon, twist slightly and stick a cocktail stick (toothpick) through the top. Make another parcel in the same way. Serve with a wedge of lemon or lime on the side.

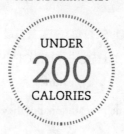

UNDER

200

CALORIES

Frozen berry smoothie

153 calories

Smoothies are excellent to have for breakfast as they are full of goodness. This recipe uses frozen berries, which makes the smoothie thick and creamy.

Serves 1   Preparation time: 2 minutes

100ml (scant ½ cup) unsweetened orange juice (18 cals)
½ banana (459 cals)
100g (3½oz) mixed berries (blackberries, raspberries, grapes, etc.), frozen (48 cals)
50g (1¾oz) low-fat plain yogurt (28 cals)

- Simply combine all the ingredients in a blender and pour into a glass.

Overnight oats

196 calories

I love this recipe, as it's tasty, filling and endlessly variable. You can prepare the ingredients in a bowl, or in a jar with a screw-top lid if you want to make it portable. You make this recipe the night before and it's ready to go the next morning.

Serves 1   Preparation time: 5 minutes, plus overnight resting (optional)

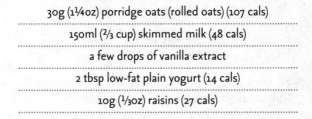

30g (1¼oz) porridge oats (rolled oats) (107 cals)

150ml (⅔ cup) skimmed milk (48 cals)

a few drops of vanilla extract

2 tbsp low-fat plain yogurt (14 cals)

10g (⅓oz) raisins (27 cals)

- Simply place all your ingredients in a bowl or jar with a screw-top lid. If it's a bowl, stir thoroughly. If it's a jar, put the lid on and shake vigorously. Leave overnight, if you like.

There are so many variations to this recipe that I couldn't possibly list them all, but here are a few to try:

Substitute the skimmed milk for water and reduce the calories (–48 cals)

OR instead of the raisins add:
10g (⅓oz) dried cranberries (32 cals)
OR
2 dried apricots, chopped (19 cals)
OR
5 almonds, chopped (61 cals)

Pink porridge

151 calories

It's called 'pink porridge' because the raspberries turn the porridge (oatmeal) a lovely pink colour. Note you can use other fresh or frozen berries to similar effect – blackberries make 'purple porridge'!

Serves 1   Preparation time: 2 minutes   Cook time: about 3 minutes

30g (1¼oz) porridge (rolled) oats (107 cals)
....
100ml (scant ½ cup) skimmed milk (32 cals)
....
50g (1¾oz) raspberries, fresh or frozen (12 cals)
....

- Place all the ingredients in a large bowl or measuring jug, pour in 100ml (scant ½ cup) water and mix together. Cook in the microwave for 3 minutes. This can also be cooked on the hob for a similar length of time.

Raisin and cranberry porridge

215 calories

Serves 1   Preparation time: 2 minutes   Cook time: about 3 minutes

30g (1¼oz) porridge (rolled) oats (107 cals)
....
100ml (scant ½ cup) skimmed milk (32 cals)
....
a few drops of vanilla extract
....
1 dessertspoon raisins (27 cals)
....
1 dessertspoon dried cranberries (49 cals)
....

- Place all the ingredients in a large bowl or measuring jug, pour in 100ml (scant ½ cup) water and cook in the microwave for 3 minutes, stirring halfway through cooking. If it is too thick, gradually add a little milk or water until it is the consistency you like. This can also be cooked on the hob for a similar length of time.

LUNCH

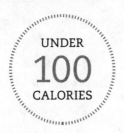

UNDER
100
CALORIES

Fresh garden soup

97 calories

This recipe makes eight portions so the rest can be frozen, if you like, for your next fast days.

Serves 8   Preparation time: 10 minutes   Cook time: about 1 hour

1 tsp olive oil (27 cals)

1 large onion, peeled and chopped (72 cals)

2 garlic cloves, peeled and finely sliced (6 cals)

2 leeks, trimmed and cut into fine rings (52 cals)

2 carrots, peeled and chopped into large chunks
(58 cals)

1 small swede (rutabaga), peeled and chopped into large
chunks (44 cals)

1 sweet potato, peeled and chopped into large chunks
(124 cals)

1 × 400g (14oz) can chopped tomatoes (72 cals)

1 tbsp tomato purée (paste) (30 cals)

continued

2 bay leaves

1 handful of fresh coriander (cilantro) stalks, roughly chopped (optional)

1 chicken or vegetable stock cube (35 cals)

80g (3¼oz) frozen peas (53 cals)

1 x 400g (14oz) can cannellini beans, drained and rinsed (210 cals)

salt and freshly ground black pepper

- Heat the olive oil in a medium-sized lidded saucepan, add the onion and garlic and fry very gently for 5 minutes. Add the leek, carrots, swede (rutabaga) and sweet potato and stir well.
- Add the canned tomatoes, tomato purée (paste), bay leaves and coriander (cilantro) stalks to the pan, then crumble in the stock cube. Top up with about 1 litre (4 cups) water. Bring the mixture to the boil, cover with a lid, then reduce the heat and simmer very gently on the lowest heat for 45 minutes. Add the peas and cannellini beans and simmer for a further 5 minutes or until the peas are cooked. Season with salt and pepper to taste and serve.

Roasted pak choi
98 calories

Roasted pak choi tastes so delicious it barely needs any accompaniment.

Serves 1   Preparation time: 2 minutes   Cook time: 8 minutes

200g (7oz) pak choi (2 large or 4 small) (38 cals)

1 tsp sesame oil (27 cals)

1 tsp olive oil (27 cals)

salt and freshly ground black pepper

1 tbsp good-quality dark soy sauce (6 cals)

continued

- Preheat the oven to 230°C/210°C fan/450°F/Gas mark 8.
- If the pak choi is large, cut in half lengthways. Place the pak choi on a baking tray and drizzle both oils over the top, then season with a pinch of salt and pepper. Bake in the oven for 7–8 minutes until tender with wilted and caramelized leaves.
- Serve the pak choi with a small dish of soy sauce on the side for dipping.

Slim spaghetti with cherry tomatoes, spinach and balsamic

92 calories

Slim spaghetti is a carbohydrate-free spaghetti that you can buy from health food shops. It may not be everyone's cup of tea, but it can be helpful when you want a 'proper' plate of food for less than 100 calories. Don't be put off by the weird smell when you first get it out of the packet; rinse the spaghetti thoroughly in warm water and the smell will disappear.

Serves 1   Preparation time: 10 minutes   Cook time: 10 minutes

100g (3½oz) slim spaghetti (8 cals)

½ tsp olive oil (14 cals)

½ garlic clove, peeled and crushed (2 cals)

10 cherry tomatoes, cut into quarters (23 cals)

50g (1¾oz) baby leaf spinach (12 cals)

freshly ground black pepper

1 tbsp good-quality balsamic vinegar (12 cals)

1 fresh basil leaf, torn

5g (⅛oz) Parmesan cheese, finely grated, to serve (21 cals)

continued

- Cook the slim spaghetti according to the packet instructions.
- Heat the olive oil in a wide saucepan over a medium heat, add the garlic and fry for 1 minute until just cooked. Add the cherry tomatoes, stir well and cook for 4 minutes. Add the spinach to the pan, stir, cover with a lid and cook for a further 1 minute. Uncover, stir in the slim spaghetti and season well with pepper. Stir in the balsamic vinegar and cook through for 1 minute. Add the torn basil and serve with a little Parmesan sprinkled over.

Basic salad
65 calories

A large bowl of salad makes a perfect fasting day meal, but there are so many variations, how do you make it work for you and how do you know how many calories there are in a salad?

A 100g (3½oz) serving of lettuce rarely has more than 15 calories, likewise a good portion of cucumber (5cm/2in) has about 10 calories. Tomatoes have a little more, with 44 calories for 2 medium tomatoes. Alternatively, 10 cherry tomatoes have 22 calories. Adding ½ a medium red (bell) pepper adds 26 calories, and 2 spring onions (scallions) add 9 calories. You can probably be safe with a calorie count of 70 for a no-frills salad without any dressing.

Serves 1   Preparation time: 5 minutes

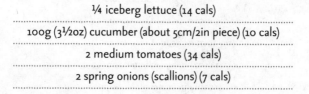

| ¼ iceberg lettuce (14 cals) |
| 100g (3½oz) cucumber (about 5cm/2in piece) (10 cals) |
| 2 medium tomatoes (34 cals) |
| 2 spring onions (scallions) (7 cals) |

- Shred the lettuce and chop the cucumber and tomatoes into rough squares. Trim the spring onions (scallions) and cut into fine rings. Add in any extras and a dressing according to the variations below, if you like.

Salad variations

Here are some easy salad extras with their respective calorie counts:

1 slice ham (41 cals)

OR

½ cooked chicken breast, shredded (115 cals)

OR

25g (1oz) mature (sharp) Cheddar cheese (103 cals)

OR

1 large egg – try boiled and sliced or poached (89 cals)

OR

2 reduced-fat bacon rashers (slices) (65 cals)

OR

2 slices pastrami (32 cals)

OR

20g (¾oz) chorizo – finely chopped for maximum flavour (58 cals)

OR

100g (3½oz) low-fat cottage cheese (79 cals)

Fat-free salad dressing

14 calories

If you want a dressing that perks up your salad without the calories then try this one.

Serves 1   Preparation time: 5 minutes, plus 5 minutes resting

2 tsp mirin (rice wine) (8 cals)
1 tbsp white wine vinegar (3 cals)
¼ tsp English mustard (3 cals)
salt and freshly ground black pepper
fresh herbs, such as basil or oregano, are a great addition but not essential

- Mix all the ingredients together in a small bowl. Leave to stand for 5 minutes to allow the flavours to develop, then drizzle the dressing over the salad.

Lemon vinaigrette salad dressing

34 calories

This is a classic salad dressing. It isn't too calorific if you keep a close watch on the amount of oil.

Serves 1   Preparation time: 2 minutes

1 lemon (2 cals)
1 tsp extra-virgin olive oil (27 cals)
1 tsp good-quality balsamic vinegar (5 cals)
salt and freshly ground black pepper
chopped fresh basil leaves (optional)

continued

- Wash the lemon in hot soapy water (only if waxed) and dry on kitchen paper (paper towels). Using the fine side of the grater, grate a little of the zest of the lemon into a small bowl, then squeeze in the juice of half of the lemon. Add the olive oil, balsamic vinegar, salt and pepper, and basil, if using. Stir, then leave to stand for 5 minutes to allow the flavours to develop before drizzling over the salad.

Honey and mustard dressing
24 calories

This dressing goes particularly well if you are adding cold meat such as chicken or ham to your salad.

Serves 1   Preparation time: 2 minutes

1 tbsp white wine vinegar (3 cals)
1 tsp runny honey (8 cals)
1 tsp wholegrain mustard (8 cals)
1 tsp balsamic vinegar (5 cals)

- Simply mix all the ingredients together and drizzle over the salad.

Creamy salad dressing

54 calories

Using low-fat yogurt here gives the dressing a creamier texture and keeps the calorie count relatively low. If you don't have any rice vinegar, then use white wine vinegar instead.

Serves 1   Preparation time: 2 minutes, plus 5 minutes resting

1 tsp very low-fat mayonnaise (29 cals)

1 tbsp low-fat plain yogurt (22 cals)

1 tbsp rice wine vinegar (3 cals)

½ tsp dried mixed herbs

salt and freshly ground black pepper

- In a small bowl, mix all the ingredients together and leave to stand for at least 5 minutes to allow the flavours to develop before drizzling over a salad.

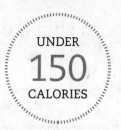

UNDER
150
CALORIES

Caesar salad dressing

106 calories

This dressing has more oomph than the average salad dressing. Serve over a salad made from romaine lettuce, cherry tomatoes and half a cooked chicken breast to make a delicious Caesar salad. If you don't have anchovy fillets, you can still make the dressing; it's not a Caesar salad dressing, but it is still definitely tasty.

Serves 1   Preparation time: 5 minutes, plus 10 minutes resting

1 anchovy fillet (7 cals)
½ garlic clove, peeled and crushed (2 cals)
1 rounded tbsp (25ml) extra-light mayonnaise (72 cals)
juice of ½ lemon (2 cals)
5g (¼oz) Parmesan cheese, finely grated (23 cals)
freshly ground black pepper

- Drain the anchovy fillet on kitchen paper (paper towels) and finely chop. Put the anchovy into a small bowl, add the garlic and use a fork to crush them together to make a rough paste. Add the mayonnaise, lemon juice, 1 tablespoon water and half the grated Parmesan. Leave to stand for about 10 minutes to allow the flavours to infuse while you prepare the salad. Mix the dressing into the salad before sprinkling over the rest of the grated Parmesan and seasoning with some pepper.

Miso broth with shiitake mushrooms

117 calories

This soup is filling, satisfying and easy to make in about 10 minutes.

Serves 1   Preparation time: 5 minutes   Cook time: 5 minutes

1 heaped tbsp miso soup paste (35 cals)

1 tsp mirin (rice wine) (14 cals)

1 tbsp dark soy sauce, plus extra for drizzling (4 cals)

1 tsp nam pla (Thai fish sauce) (4 cals)

1cm (½in) piece fresh root ginger, peeled and grated (5 cals)

50g (1¾oz) spring greens or Savoy cabbage,
thinly sliced (14 cals)

½ carrot, peeled and cut into very fine batons (13 cals)

50g (1¾oz) beansprouts (16 cals)

50g (1¾oz) shiitake mushrooms, sliced (12 cals)

- Bring 500ml (generous 2 cups) water to boiling point in a large saucepan. Stir in the miso soup paste, mirin, soy, nam pla and ginger, then add the greens, carrot, beansprouts and mushrooms and simmer gently for 5 minutes.
- Serve in a wide bowl with soy sauce drizzled over the top.

Mushroom stir-fry

146 calories

This is a filling and substantial stir-fry, yet it is low in calories too.

Serves 1　Preparation time: 5 minutes　Cook time: 6 minutes

½ tsp walnut oil (20 cals)

1 tbsp dark soy sauce (6 cals)

1 tsp soft dark brown sugar (18 cals)

½ tsp sunflower oil (14 cals)

½ garlic clove, peeled and finely chopped (2 cals)

½ yellow (bell) pepper, deseeded and cut into
thin slices (21 cals)

½ small carrot, peeled and cut into very thin sticks
(14 cals)

1 small thumb fresh root ginger, peeled and cut
into very thin sticks (6 cals)

50g (1¾oz) beansprouts (16 cals)

50g (1¾oz) mangetout (snow peas) (16 cals)

100g (3½oz) mushrooms, sliced (13 cals)

- In a bowl, mix together the walnut oil, soy sauce and brown sugar to make a sauce.
- Heat the oil in a wok or large frying pan (skillet) over a high heat, toss in the garlic, (bell) pepper, carrot and ginger and stir-fry for 2 minutes. Add the beansprouts, mangetout (snow peas) and mushrooms and stir-fry for a further 2 minutes. Reduce the heat to medium, add the sauce and cook for another 2 minutes. Serve immediately.

Stuffed courgette rolls

121 calories

In this delicious Italian starter (appetizer) the thin slices of courgette (zucchini) are 'cooked' in oil and vinegar before being stuffed with a delicious cottage cheese filling. This recipe makes four or five rolls.

Serves 1   Preparation time: 5 minutes, plus at least 20 minutes marinating

1 courgette (zucchini) (18 cals)

1 tsp extra-virgin olive oil (27 cals)

1 tbsp balsamic vinegar (12 cals)

100g (3½oz) low-fat cottage cheese (63 cals)

1 tsp lemon juice (1 cal)

4 fresh basil leaves, shredded

salt and freshly ground black pepper

- Cut the ends off the courgette (zucchini) and, using a vegetable peeler, cut 4 long strips, discarding the first and last strips that are just skin.
- Drizzle the olive oil and half the balsamic vinegar over a large plate. Arrange the courgette strips flat on the plate, making sure they don't overlap, then drizzle the remaining balsamic vinegar over the top. Leave to marinate in the refrigerator for at least 20 minutes.
- Place the cottage cheese in a fine sieve (strainer) and press on it gently with a fork to remove as much liquid as possible. Put the cottage cheese into a small bowl and mix in the lemon juice and shredded basil, then season.
- Place 1 generous teaspoon of the cottage cheese mixture onto one end of a courgette strip and roll up. Repeat until you have used up all the filling. Arrange the rolls upright on a serving plate to serve.

Fragrant chicken broth

122 calories

This tasty broth somehow manages to be both fresh and warming at the same time. Warning: this is quite hot and spicy, so if you don't like it too hot, use just one chilli. This broth serves four, so make the whole quantity and freeze three portions for your next fast days.

Serves 4   Preparation time: 5 minutes   Cook time: about 30 minutes

1 litre (4 cups) fresh chicken stock (70 cals)
2 green chillies, deseeded and chopped into rings (2 cals)
6 spring onions (scallions), trimmed and shredded (55 cals)
1 thumb fresh root ginger, peeled and cut into very thin strips (9 cals)
1 red (bell) pepper, deseeded and cut into strips (51 cals)
2 limes (5 cals)
a pinch of ground mace
1 tsp salt
1 tsp nam pla (Thai fish sauce) (4 cals)
1 tsp rice vinegar
1 × 400ml (14fl oz) can reduced-fat coconut milk (292 cals)

- Heat the chicken stock with the chillies, spring onions (scallions), ginger and red (bell) pepper. Using a fine grater, grate in the zest of 1 lime. Add a pinch of mace, the salt, nam pla and rice vinegar and simmer for 20 minutes. Juice the limes.
- Stir in the coconut milk and lime juice, and heat for a further 5 minutes until hot and just bubbling. Serve immediately.
- If you like you can add extra ingredients such as mushrooms (13 calories for 100g/3½oz) or green beans (35 calories for 100g/3½oz).

Prawn and plum kebabs

112 calories

You can use either metal or wooden skewers here, but if using wooden ones remember to soak them in a bowl of cold water for at least 30 minutes before using, otherwise they may burn during cooking.

Serves 1   Preparation time: 5 minutes   Cook time: 8 minutes

1 tsp olive oil (7 cals)

1 tbsp chopped fresh coriander (cilantro) (1 cal)

grated zest and juice of 1 lime (4 cals)

2 slices jalapeño peppers in brine,
chopped (4 cals)

a pinch of salt

100g (3½oz) raw king prawns (king shrimp) (76 cals)

1 fresh plum, pitted and cut into 6 pieces (20 cals)

- Combine the olive oil, coriander (cilantro), lime zest and juice, chopped jalapeños and salt in a small bowl. Set aside 2 teaspoons of the mixture to use later as a dressing.
- Place the prawns (shrimp) and plum in a bowl, add the marinade and toss to coat.
- Preheat the grill (broiler) to medium-high.
- Thread the prawns and plums alternately onto 2 skewers, then place on the grill pan and grill (broil) for 3–4 minutes on each side until they are opaque and a little caramelized at the edges. Serve with the reserved dressing drizzled over.

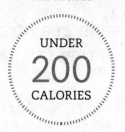

Mozzarella and tomato salad

166 calories

Serves 1   Preparation time: 5 minutes

1 tsp extra-virgin olive oil (27 cals)

1 tsp good-quality balsamic vinegar (2 cals)

salt and freshly ground black pepper

½ ball light Italian mozzarella (95 cals)

1 beef (beefsteak) tomato (42 cals)

6 fresh basil leaves

- First, make the dressing. Mix the olive oil, balsamic vinegar and salt and pepper to taste together and set aside.
- Cut the mozzarella into 6 thin slices and cut the tomato into 6 slices.
- Starting on one side of a serving plate, place a slice of tomato, followed by a slice of mozzarella and finally a basil leaf. They should be overlapping a little and starting to cross the plate. Continue layering in this order – tomato, mozzarella and basil – until there is 6 of each.
- When you are ready to serve, drizzle the dressing along the central line of the salad.

Sugar snap pea, mint and barley salad

165 calories

You can buy pearl barley in health food stores and most supermarkets. A much underused grain, it goes particularly well with the crunchy sugar snap peas in this healthy salad.

Serves 1   Preparation time: 10 minutes   Cook time: about 35 minutes

25g (1oz) pearl barley, rinsed (90 cals)

100g (3½oz) sugar snap peas, trimmed and cut into diagonal strips (34 cals)

1 tbsp chopped fresh flat-leaf (Italian) parsley

1 tsp chopped fresh mint

¼ red onion, peeled and finely chopped (12 cals)

1 tsp extra-virgin olive oil (27 cals)

juice of ½ lemon (2 cals)

salt and freshly ground black pepper

- Cook the barley in a pan of water for 20–30 minutes, until tender. Pearl barley can have varied cooking times, so always check the packet instructions and cook the barley for the length of time suggested.
- Rinse the barley in cool water and transfer to a bowl. Add the sugar snap peas, parsley, mint and onion and toss to combine.
- Mix the olive oil, lemon juice and salt and pepper to taste in a small bowl to make a dressing, then pour over the salad and serve.

Cajun roasted vegetables

175 calories

This is a great way to use up vegetables you have in the refrigerator. Roasting in cajun spices brings new life to practically any veg.

Serves 1   Preparation time: 10 minutes   Cook time: about 25 minutes

1 tsp olive oil (27 cals)

2 tsp cajun spices

2 garlic cloves, unpeeled (6 cals)

1 red onion, peeled and cut into eighths lengthways (40 cals)

6 small cauliflower florets (18 cals)

6 baby carrots (24 cals)

6 baby corns (22 cals)

1 leek, trimmed and cut into thick rings (38 cals)

- Preheat the oven to 220°C/fan 200°C/425°F/Gas mark 7.
- In a large bowl, combine the olive oil, cajun spices, garlic and 2 tablespoons water. Add the vegetables to the bowl and toss thoroughly. It's best to use your hands. Transfer the vegetables to a roasting dish and roast in the oven for 20–25 minutes until cooked.
- Remove the vegetables from the oven and use a fork to squash the garlic cloves firmly, releasing their garlicky juices. Mix the vegetables again with a metal spoon and serve.

Roasted sweet potato with quick-cook chilli vegetables

183 calories

This has to be one of my favourite easy lunches for one.

Serves 1   Cook time: 45 minutes (potato), 10 minutes (chilli)

1 small sweet potato (about 100g/3½oz) (87 cals)

½ tsp olive oil (14 cals)

1 yellow (bell) pepper, roughly diced (42 cals)

½ garlic clove, peeled and finely chopped (2 cals)

1 spring onion (scallion), cut into fine rings (5 cals)

salt and freshly ground black pepper

¼ tsp ground cumin

½ tsp mild chilli powder

½ tsp paprika (3 cal)

1 tbsp tomato purée (paste) (30 cals)

- Preheat the oven to 200°C/fan 180°C/400°F/Gas mark 6.
- Prick the sweet potato all over with a fork and roast in the oven for 30–45 minutes, depending on size. If you want to speed up the roasting process, cook on full power in the microwave for 2–3 minutes before placing in the oven.
- Meanwhile, heat the oil in a frying pan (skillet) over a medium heat, add the (bell) pepper and fry for 3 minutes. Add the garlic and spring onion (scallion) and fry for a further 2 minutes. Reduce the heat to low, add a pinch of salt and the spices, then stir and cook for a further minute. Stir in the tomato purée (paste) and 3 tablespoons water and cook gently for 5 minutes.
- Cut a deep cross in the top of the sweet potato and gently squeeze the sides to mash the potato and push it out of the top. Season with salt and pepper, spoon the chilli onto the top of the potato and eat immediately.

Stuffed pepper

187 calories

Serves 1   Preparation time: 10 minutes   Cook time: 15 minutes

1 red (bell) pepper (51 cals)
10g (⅓oz) pine nuts (69 cals)
1 tsp olive oil (27 cals)
½ garlic clove, peeled and chopped (2 cals)
100g (3½oz) mushrooms, diced (13 cals)
1 small courgette (zucchini), trimmed and diced (25 cals)
salt and freshly ground black pepper
1 tsp chopped fresh parsley, to serve

- Preheat the oven to 220°C/fan 200°C/425°F/Gas mark 7.
- Cut the (bell) pepper in half lengthways, leaving the stalk intact. Cut out under the stalk and pull out the seeds and pith. Place the pepper halves cut side down on a baking tray and cook in the oven for 10 minutes.
- Meanwhile, prepare the filling. Heat a small frying pan (skillet) over a medium heat. Add the pine nuts and toast for 2–3 minutes until browning all over. Set aside.
- Heat the olive oil in the same pan over a medium-low heat, add the garlic and fry for 1 minute. Add the mushrooms and courgette (zucchini) and fry for 5–6 minutes, stirring occasionally.
- Remove the peppers from the oven. Turn them over and leave them on the baking tray. Spoon the vegetable mixture into the pepper halves. You can squeeze the filling down a little, being careful not to break the peppers. Season with a little salt and pepper, then return the peppers to the oven and cook for a further 5 minutes.
- Serve the peppers with the toasted pine nuts and chopped parsley sprinkled over the top.

Perfect flatbread

153 calories

I have been searching for some time for the perfect flatbread recipe, as I want something low in calories that I can eat occasionally on my fast day and something that is very nutritious and tasty that I can eat on 'normal' days. This flatbread is much better than bought flatbread and has a real artisan look and taste. I have included instructions for making this by hand as well as using a bread machine.

Makes 6 flatbreads   Preparation time: 25 minutes, plus 1 hour 20 minutes resting or time in bread machine   Cook time: 4 minutes

250g (9oz) strong white bread flour, plus extra for dusting (830 cals)
¾ tsp fast-action yeast (active dry yeast) (4 cals)
1 tsp sugar (20 cals)
a pinch of salt
1 tsp olive oil (27 cals)
2 tbsp low-fat plain yogurt (39 cals)

Making the dough by hand

- Put the flour into a large mixing bowl and stir in the yeast, sugar and salt. Make a well in the centre and add the oil, yogurt and 60ml (¼ cup) water and start to bring the mixture together with your hands. Add another 60ml (¼ cup) water slowly and mix until all the flour is combined.
- Put the dough on a lightly floured work surface (counter) and knead for about 10 minutes until the dough is smooth and almost silky. Return the dough to the mixing bowl, cover and leave in a warm place for 1 hour or until the dough has doubled in size.

continued

Making the dough in a bread machine

- Put the yeast in the bottom of the bread pan and put the flour on top of that. Add the rest of the ingredients and turn the bread machine onto the 'dough' or 'basic dough' setting.

Making the flatbreads

- Line a baking sheet with greaseproof (waxed) paper.
- Tip the dough out onto a lightly floured work surface (counter) and fold repeatedly to knock the air out of it, then cut the dough into 6 equal pieces and roll each into a ball.
- Put a ball of dough on a well-floured work surface and use a rolling pin to flatten it to a circle or oval of about 15cm (6in) wide. Place it on the prepared baking sheet and repeat with the remaining dough. You should be able to squeeze 3 flatbreads onto a standard-sized baking sheet. Place the baking sheets in a warm place to rest for 20 minutes.
- Heat a large frying pan (skillet) over a medium-high heat and, when hot, place 2 flatbreads into the pan, pushing them lightly against the base of the pan. Cook for 2 minutes – they should puff up and be a little blackened and blistered in places. Turn them over and cook for another 2 minutes. Remove and wrap in a clean tea towel (dish towel) while you cook the other flatbreads.
- These flatbreads are at their absolute best served immediately, but it you want to reheat them in the oven, sprinkle with water and cook in an oven preheated to 220°C/fan 200°C/425°F/Gas mark 7 for 4–5 minutes until hot.
- I have listed several toppings and fillings for the flatbreads on the following pages, but there are endless variations. If you fancy making one of these but don't want to make your own flatbreads, then I recommend using the shop-bought mini naan breads. They vary in calories but normally work out at around 150 calories per naan bread. Cook them according to the packet instructions.

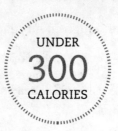

UNDER
300
CALORIES

Courgette and tomato flatbread

216 calories

Serves 1   Preparation time: 7 minutes   Cook time: about 8 minutes

½ tsp olive oil (14 cals)

1 medium courgette (zucchini), trimmed and diced (27 cals)

10 cherry tomatoes, cut into quarters (22 cals)

salt and freshly ground black pepper

- Heat the olive oil in a pan, add the courgette (zucchini) and tomatoes and gently fry for 5–6 minutes. Pile the courgettes and tomatoes on top of the warm flatbread and season with salt and pepper. Serve immediately.

Folded feta and olive flatbread

244 calories

Serves 1   Preparation time: 2 minutes

25g (1oz) light feta cheese, cut into cubes (45 cals)

5 large black olives, roughly chopped (26 cals)

5cm (2in) piece cucumber, diced (10 cals)

1 tbsp balsamic vinegar (10 cals)

freshly ground black pepper

- Mix all the ingredients together in a small bowl, then spoon the mixture onto half of the still warm flatbread and gently fold over. Serve immediately.

Flatbread with garlicky tomato sauce and anchovies

224 calories

Serves 1   Preparation time: 5 minutes   Cook time: about 8 minutes

½ tsp extra-virgin olive oil (14 cals)

1 garlic clove, peeled and finely chopped (3 cals)

1 tbsp tomato purée (paste) (30 cals)

4 anchovy fillets, drained (24 cals)

- Heat the olive oil gently in a small frying pan (skillet), add the garlic and fry for 1–2 minutes until just starting to brown. Stir in the tomato purée (paste) and 2 tablespoons water, then fry gently for another 4–5 minutes.
- Spread the tomato sauce over a warm flatbread and arrange the anchovies over the top. Slice into quarters and eat straight away.

Chorizo and green pepper flatbread

239 calories

Serves 1   Preparation time: 5 minutes   Cook time: 5 minutes

20g (¾oz) Spanish chorizo, cut into small dice (58 cals)

1 shallot, peeled and cut into small dice (16 cals)

½ green (bell) pepper, deseeded and diced (12 cals)

- Heat a frying pan (skillet) then toss all the ingredients into the pan and fry for about 5 minutes. Serve piled on top of a hot flatbread.

Halloumi salad

215 calories

Serves 1   Preparation time: 5 minutes
Cook time: 8 minutes, plus 10 minutes cooling

2 vine-ripened tomatoes, sliced (26 cals)

½ red (bell) pepper, deseeded and cut into strips (25 cals)

50g (1¾oz) light halloumi, drained and sliced
into thin squares (122 cals)

75g (3oz) Italian mixed salad leaves (greens) (10 cals)

For the marinade:

½ garlic clove, peeled and crushed (2 cals)

juice of 1 lime (3 cals)

1 tsp chopped fresh parsley

½ tsp chilli flakes (red pepper flakes)

freshly ground black pepper

1 tsp extra-virgin olive oil (27 cals)

- To make the marinade, combine the garlic, lime juice, parsley, chilli flakes (red pepper flakes), pepper, 1 tablespoon water and the olive oil in a wide bowl.
- Add the sliced tomatoes to the marinade. Heat a large frying pan (skillet) and dry-fry the red (bell) pepper strips for about 5 minutes until slightly blackened, then put them with the tomatoes in the marinade.
- Fry the halloumi slices in the same pan until golden on both sides – they will only take a minute in a hot pan. When they are cooked, add them to the marinade and turn until the halloumi is coated all over. Leave the halloumi to cool for about 10 minutes.
- Arrange the salad leaves (greens) on a wide serving plate and put the halloumi, pepper strips and tomatoes on top. Drizzle over the remaining marinade and serve.

Tuna and bean salad

293 calories

Serves 1   Preparation time: 5 minutes, plus 20 minutes standing

¼ red onion, peeled and finely chopped (16 cals)

juice of 1 lemon (4 cals)

1 × 400g (14oz) can borlotti beans, rinsed
and drained (95 cals)

1 × 200g (7oz) can good-quality tuna in water,
drained (154 cals)

5cm (2in) piece cucumber, peeled and cut into large
chunks (10 cals)

1 small handful of fresh flat-leaf (Italian)
parsley leaves, chopped

½ tsp extra-virgin olive oil (14 cals)

salt and freshly ground black pepper

- Put the chopped onion into a bowl and stir in the lemon juice. Leave to stand for at least 10 minutes.
- Place the drained borlotti beans in a wide bowl and flake the tuna into the beans. Add the cucumber and stir through the chopped parsley.
- Add the olive oil to the onions and season with salt and pepper, then pour the onion mixture over the tuna and beans. Stir through and leave at room temperature for another 10 minutes to allow the flavours to fully develop before serving.

Yin and yang chicken salad

211 calories

This Asian-style salad should keep you going through the day.

Serves 2 Preparation time: 30 minutes Cook time: about 15 minutes

220g (7½oz) skinless, boneless chicken breast,
cut into strips (233 cals)

½ onion, peeled and roughly chopped (27 cals)

1 bay leaf

1 stalk lemongrass, bruised with the back of a knife

For the salad:

100g (3½oz) cucumber (5cm/2in piece), peeled (10 cals)

a pinch of salt

1 celery stick, cut into long, thin strips (5 cals)

1 medium carrot, peeled and cut into
long, thin strips (35 cals)

80g (3¼oz) white cabbage, thinly shredded (22 cals)

1 small handful of fresh coriander (cilantro) leaves,
roughly chopped (3 cals)

1 small handful of fresh mint leaves,
roughly chopped (6 cals)

2 tsp sesame seeds (60 cals)

6 little gem lettuce leaves (3 cals)

continued

For the dressing:

½ garlic clove, peeled and crushed (2 cals)

½ small red chilli, deseeded and cut into rings (1 cal)

½ tsp granulated sugar (10 cals)

juice of 1 lime (4 cals)

1 tsp fish sauce (1 cal)

salt and freshly ground black pepper

- Place the chicken in a lidded saucepan and add the onion, bay leaf and lemongrass. Cover with water and bring to the boil. Put the lid on the pan, reduce the heat and simmer for 10–12 minutes or until the chicken is cooked. Remove the chicken from the pan with a slotted spoon and leave to cool.
- For the salad, using a vegetable peeler, cut the cucumber into flat strips. Discard the seeds, then place on a large plate and sprinkle with the salt. Set aside for 10 minutes.
- Meanwhile, make the dressing by placing all the dressing ingredients in a small bowl, adding 1 tablespoon water and mixing together.
- Squeeze the excess water out of the cucumber, then place in a large bowl and add the celery, carrot, cabbage and herbs. Mix in the cooked chicken and half the sesame seeds, then stir in the dressing.
- Arrange the lettuce leaves on 2 serving plates, then pile the salad on top of the lettuce and sprinkle with the remaining sesame seeds. Serve.

Roasted red pepper couscous

216 calories

Prepare this salad a little differently, by dressing the couscous before it's rehydrated. You also 'cook' the couscous in cold water so it retains a satisfying bite.

Serves 1   Preparation time: 10 minutes, plus 20 minutes standing

Cook time: 20 minutes

1 red (bell) pepper, whole (51 cals)
1 tsp extra-virgin olive oil (27 cals)
½ tsp English mustard (6 cals)
1 tbsp white wine vinegar (1 cal)
½ tsp granulated sugar (8 cals)
salt and freshly ground black pepper
1 tsp chopped fresh coriander (cilantro) leaves
1 tsp chopped fresh basil leaves
40g (1½oz) couscous, uncooked (91 cals)
10 cherry tomatoes, cut into quarters (22 cals)
100g (3½oz) cucumber, peeled and diced (10 cals)

- Preheat the oven to 200°C/fan 180°C/400°F/Gas mark 6.
- Place the red (bell) pepper on a baking sheet and roast in the oven for 20 minutes.
- Meanwhile, make a dressing by mixing the olive oil, mustard, vinegar, sugar, salt and pepper to taste and herbs together in a small bowl.
- Place the couscous in a bowl, then pour over the dressing and mix lightly with a fork. Leave to stand for 5 minutes, then pour over enough water just to cover the couscous and leave for a further 15 minutes until the couscous has absorbed the water. Fluff the couscous up with a fork.

continued

- When the pepper is cooked, take out of the oven and remove and discard the stalk and seeds. Remove any loose pieces of skin, then chop the pepper flesh into cubes and add to the couscous together with the tomatoes and cucumber. Serve immediately or keep in the refrigerator for up to two days.

Stuffed avocado
284 calories

Avocados have a lot of calories, but they are very healthy and tasty too.

Serves 1 Preparation time: 5 minutes

1 medium ripe avocado (250 cals)
6 cherry tomatoes, cut into quarters (14 cals)
100g (3½oz) cucumber (5cm/2in piece), peeled and cut into small cubes (10 cals)
2 tsp good-quality balsamic vinegar (10 cals)
salt and freshly ground black pepper

- Prepare the avocado by cutting it in half and removing the stone (pit). Mix the tomatoes, cucumber and vinegar together in a small bowl, then season with salt and pepper and spoon over the avocados. Serve immediately.

MAIN MEALS

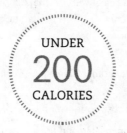

UNDER
200
CALORIES

Quick fried chickpeas with rocket

200 calories

Serves 2   Preparation time: 1 minute   Cook time: 8 minutes

1 tsp olive oil (27 cals)
1 tsp cumin seeds
1 garlic clove, peeled and finely chopped (3 cals)
1 × 400g (14oz) can chickpeas, rinsed and drained (304 cals)
a pinch of salt
1½ tbsp mirin (rice wine) (52 cals)
75g (3oz) wild rocket (arugula) (14 cals)

- Heat the olive oil in a wide frying pan (skillet), add the cumin seeds and garlic and fry for 1–2 minutes until the garlic is just starting to turn brown. Add the chickpeas, salt and mirin (rice wine), stir well and cook for a further 4 minutes. Add the rocket (arugula) and stir gently for 2 minutes or until the rocket has wilted. Serve immediately.

Red lentil dal

196 calories

This filling dish freezes really well, so make a big pot and freeze some for a speedy dinner another day. This dal can be eaten on its own or with basmati rice, chapatti or a flatbread.

Serves 4   Preparation time: 10 minutes   Cook time: about 1 hour

1 tbsp sunflower oil (99 cals)
1 large onion, peeled and finely chopped (86 cals)
4 garlic cloves, peeled and finely chopped (12 cals)
2.5cm (1in) piece fresh root ginger, peeled and grated (5 cals)
1 large red chilli, deseeded and chopped into fine rings (3 cals)
¼ tsp ground turmeric
¼ tsp cayenne pepper
1 tsp paprika (7 cals)
½ tsp ground cumin
a pinch of salt
180g (6½oz) dried red lentils, rinsed (572 cals)
juice of 2 limes (7 cals)
1 tomato, finely chopped (14 cals)

- Heat the oil in a heavy-based pan over a low-medium heat. Add the onion, garlic, ginger and chilli and stir-fry for 3–4 minutes. Add the ground spices and salt and stir-fry for another minute. Add the lentils, stir, then pour in 900ml (3½ cups) water and bring to the boil. Reduce the heat slightly and simmer vigorously for 10 minutes, then reduce the heat to low and cook for a further 35–40 minutes, stirring regularly, until all the water has been

continued

absorbed. If the dal is too thick or starts to stick on the base of the pan, just add a little more water. When the dal has the consistency of thick porridge, add the lime juice and tomato and cook for a further 3 minutes before serving.

Coriander and lemon chicken
199 calories

This chicken dish is incredibly fresh and tasty. Serve with a zingy salad.

Serves 1   Preparation time: 5 minutes, plus 1 hour marinating
Cook time: 15 minutes

1 × 150g (5oz) skinless, boneless chicken breast, cut in half and scored lightly with a knife (159 cals)
½ lemon (8 cals)
½ garlic clove, peeled and crushed (2 cals)
1 handful of fresh coriander (cilantro) leaves, chopped (4 cals)
1 tsp olive oil (27 cals)
salt and freshly ground black pepper

- Put the chicken into the marinade and use your fingers to rub the marinade all over until the chicken is coated. Cover and leave to rest in the refrigerator for at least 1 hour.
- Wash the lemon in hot soapy water (only if waxed) and dry on kitchen paper (paper towels). Using the fine side of the grater, grate a little of the zest of the lemon into a medium-sized bowl. Add the garlic, coriander (cilantro) leaves, olive oil and the juice of the ½ lemon. Mix together with a little salt and pepper.
- Heat a griddle pan or frying pan (skillet) over a medium-high heat. Add the chicken, press it into the pan and cook for about 6–8 minutes on each side, turning the heat down if it looks like it's starting to catch, until the chicken is cooked through. Leave to rest in the pan for 2 minutes before serving.

Honey mustard chicken skewers

200 calories

The chicken in this dish is very tender and delicious. Serve with a green salad, adding on the appropriate calories if you are on a fast day. If using wooden skewers, make sure they are soaked in a bowl of water for at least 30 minutes before using to prevent them burning during cooking.

Serves 1   Preparation time: 5 minutes,
plus 30 minutes marinating (optional)   Cook time: 16 minutes

2 tsp wholegrain mustard (14 cals)

1 tsp runny honey (23 cals)

grated zest and juice of 1 lime (4 cals)

1 x 150g (5oz) skinless, boneless chicken breast, cut into
6 small pieces (159 cals)

- Mix the mustard, honey, lime zest and juice and 1 tablespoon water together in a bowl. Add the chicken and stir until the chicken pieces are coated all over with the marinade. You could cook the chicken straight away but it tastes much better if it is left to marinate for about 30 minutes in the refrigerator.
- Preheat the grill (broiler) to medium. Thread the chicken pieces onto skewers. You want 2 short skewers with 3 pieces of chicken on each, leaving room between the chicken pieces to allow them to cook thoroughly.
- Place the chicken skewers on a grill pan and grill (broil) for 6–8 minutes on each side. Check that the chicken is cooked through and chargrilled all over before serving.

Haddock tapenade

158 calories

This is a light and healthy supper for one. Serve on a bed of green beans or wilted spinach.

Serves 1   Preparation time: 2 minutes   Cook time: 17 minutes

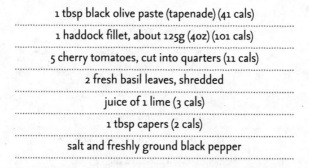

1 tbsp black olive paste (tapenade) (41 cals)
1 haddock fillet, about 125g (4oz) (101 cals)
5 cherry tomatoes, cut into quarters (11 cals)
2 fresh basil leaves, shredded
juice of 1 lime (3 cals)
1 tbsp capers (2 cals)
salt and freshly ground black pepper

- Spread the olive paste on both sides of the fish. Heat a non-stick frying pan (skillet) over a medium heat, place the haddock in the pan and cook for 10–15 minutes, turning once. The cooking time depends on the thickness of the fillet. Transfer the fish to a warm plate.
- Add the tomatoes, basil, lime juice and capers to the pan and heat gently for 2 minutes before pouring over the haddock. Season with salt and pepper to taste before serving.

Baked fish parcel

197 calories

Cooking fish and vegetables in a foil parcel is not only tasty but very healthy for your fast day. I use cod, but any firm white fish would work well. Serve over wilted spinach.

Serves 1   Preparation time: 5 minutes   Cook time: about 20 minutes

1 small boneless, skinless cod fillet (about 100g/3½oz) (80 cals)
4 spring onions (scallions), trimmed but left whole (28 cals)
100ml (scant ½ cup) white wine (66 cals)
½ garlic clove, peeled and finely sliced (2 cals)
1 tsp wholegrain mustard (7 cals)
½ tsp extra-virgin olive oil (14 cals)
½ tsp dried mixed herbs or fresh oregano or basil
salt and freshly ground black pepper

- Preheat the oven to 220°C/fan200°C/425°F/Gas mark 7.
- First make a foil parcel using two sheets of foil. Each sheet should be roughly square, using the standard width of the foil as one side. Place the two sheets one on top of the other and fold the top sheet in so it makes a rather flat shoebox shape with an open top. You will be putting the fish and other ingredients in the shoebox, so make sure it will hold liquid without falling apart.
- Put the fish inside the foil and arrange the spring onions (scallions) around it.
- In a small bowl, mix together the wine, garlic, mustard, olive oil and herbs. Pour over the fish and season well with salt and pepper. Seal the parcel by bringing up the edges of the outer layer of foil and rolling over to make a loose seal. You should leave plenty of air above the fish rather than make a tight parcel as this will allow steam to circulate. Place the parcel on a baking tray and cook in the oven for 18–20 minutes. Serve immediately, being careful when you open the parcel as hot steam will escape.

White fish with sweet chilli and ginger sauce

140 calories

This simple supper can be prepared and cooked in 10 minutes. Serve with seasonal green vegetables or new potatoes if you are feeling decadent!

Serves 1   Preparation time: 2 minutes   Cook time: about 8 minutes

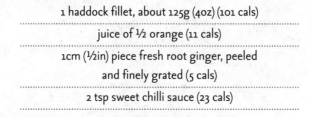

1 haddock fillet, about 125g (4oz) (101 cals)
juice of ½ orange (11 cals)
1cm (½in) piece fresh root ginger, peeled and finely grated (5 cals)
2 tsp sweet chilli sauce (23 cals)

- Cut the haddock in half lengthways so you have 2 thin fillets.
- Heat a non-stick frying pan (skillet) over a medium heat, add the haddock and cook for 4–5 minutes on each side. When the haddock is just cooked, turn the heat down to low, squeeze in the orange juice then add the ginger and sweet chilli sauce. Stir gently so it is all mixed together but without disturbing the fish. Turn the fish over so it is completely coated in the sauce and heat for 2 minutes until warmed through. Serve immediately.

Tandoori mixed fish grill

154 calories

I have used trout, salmon and prawns (shrimp) in this grill, but feel free to substitute any white fish for the salmon, if you prefer.

Serves 4   Preparation time: 5 minutes, plus 1–2 hours marinating
Cook time: 16 minutes

continued

1 skinless trout fillet, about 100g (3½oz) (125 cals)

1 skinless salmon fillet, about 130g (4½oz) (234 cals)

225g (8oz) raw king prawns (king shrimp) (171 cals)

lemon wedges, to serve

For the marinade:

4 tbsp low-fat plain yogurt (78 cals)

grated zest of 1 lemon

2.5cm (1in) piece fresh root ginger, peeled and
finely grated (5 cals)

1 garlic clove, peeled and finely grated (3 cals)

½ tsp ground cumin

½ tsp chilli powder

¼ tsp turmeric

¼ tsp garam masala

a pinch of salt

- Mix all the marinade ingredients together in a small bowl.
- Cut the trout and salmon into 4 pieces each, then place the trout, salmon and prawns (shrimp) in a plastic bag and spoon in the marinade. Make sure that all the fish is coated in the marinade. Seal and leave to marinate in the refrigerator for 1–2 hours.
- Preheat the grill (broiler) to medium or light the barbecue. Put the salmon and trout pieces under the grill and cook for 6–8 minutes on each side. They should be brown and crispy and cooked through. Towards the end of the cooking time add the prawns as they only need 1–2 minutes each side, otherwise they will go rubbery.
- Serve on a bed of crispy salad leaves (100g/3½oz = 16 cals) with lemon wedges on the side.

Homemade fish fingers with lemon mayo

180 calories

This recipe makes four servings, but the fish fingers can be frozen before they are cooked, then cooked from frozen – just add an extra 10 minutes to the cooking time.

Serves 4   Preparation time: 10 minutes   Cook time: 15–18 minutes

1 tbsp olive oil (99 cals)
1 egg, beaten (76 cals)
80g (3¼oz) white breadcrumbs (175 cals)
½ tsp dried mixed herbs
grated zest and juice of 1 lemon (3 cals)
salt and freshly ground black pepper
400g (14oz) white fish (cod, haddock, pollack, etc.), cut into 12 strips (320 cals)
4 tbsp extra-light mayonnaise (48 cals)

- Preheat the oven to 220°C/fan 200°C/425°F/Gas mark 7. Brush a non-stick baking tray with a little of the olive oil.
- Pour the beaten egg into a wide bowl. Put the breadcrumbs on a plate, add in the mixed herbs, lemon zest and a little salt and pepper, and combine.
- Dip each piece of fish first in the egg, then in the breadcrumbs, making sure it's lightly coated in each, and put on the prepared baking tray. Lightly drizzle the remaining olive oil over the top and cook in the oven for 15–18 minutes until golden.
- Meanwhile, mix the mayonnaise and lemon juice together in a small bowl.
- Serve the fish goujons with the lemon mayonnaise on the side.

Barbecued tiger prawns with saffron aïoli

167 calories

These prawns (shrimp) are delicious served with a green salad. Add on the appropriate calories if you are on a fast day.

Serves 2   Preparation time: 5 minutes, plus 1 hour marinating
Cook time: 4 minutes

225g (8oz) raw tiger prawns (jumbo shrimp) (171 cals)

juice of ½ lemon (2 cals)

For the marinade:

2 garlic cloves, peeled and finely chopped (6 cals)

grated zest of 1 lemon

1 tbsp olive oil (99 cals)

1 tsp finely chopped fresh parsley

salt and freshly ground black pepper

For the aïoli:

juice of ½ lemon (2 cals)

½ tsp saffron threads

½ garlic clove, peeled and finely chopped (2 cals)

2 tbsp white wine (22 cals)

2 tbsp extra-light mayonnaise (30 cals)

- To make the marinade, mix the garlic, lemon zest, olive oil, parsley and salt and pepper to taste together in a large bowl. Add the prawns (shrimp) and coat well with the marinade. Leave to marinate in the refrigerator for at least 1 hour.

- To make the aïoli, place the lemon juice, saffron, garlic and white wine in a saucepan. Bring to the boil, then reduce the heat and simmer for 5 minutes. Place the mayonnaise in a bowl, pour in the lemon juice mixture and stir well.
- When you are ready to cook the prawns, light the barbecue or preheat the grill (broiler) to high, then grill (broil) the prawns for 1–2 minutes on each side until cooked through. Pile the prawns in a bowl and squeeze the lemon juice over the top. Serve with the aïoli on the side.

My favourite curry sauce
186 calories

This is my ultimate favourite curry – fast day or not. Don't be put off by the list of spices, as it is totally worth it. I have included three versions, with mushrooms, vegetables and chicken, so you can match the recipe to your needs (see pages 134, 155 and 156).

Serves 2 Preparation time: 30 minutes Cook time: 30 minutes

For the paste:

2 tsp coriander seeds
1 tsp cumin seeds
4 cardamom pods
8 black peppercorns
4 cloves
1 tbsp desiccated (dry unsweetened) coconut (60 cals)
2.5cm (1in) piece fresh root ginger, peeled and grated (9 cals)
6 garlic cloves, peeled and grated (18 cals)
1 tsp sunflower oil (27 cals)
2 tsp ground almonds (92 cals)

continued

¾ tsp salt

½ tsp mild chilli powder

¼ tsp turmeric

For the curry sauce:

a few sprays of 1 cal oil (3 cals)

1 small onion, peeled and finely chopped (40 cals)

2 bird's eye (Thai) chillies, deseeded and chopped into rings

3 tbsp low-fat plain yogurt (59 cals)

1 × 400g (14oz) can chopped tomatoes (64 cals)

- First, prepare the spice paste. Put the coriander seeds in a small frying pan (skillet) and heat to a high temperature until they start to pop. Set aside, then toast the cumin seeds, cardamom pods, peppercorns and cloves. When they start popping remove from the pan and set aside with the coriander seeds. Finally, toast the desiccated (dry unsweetened) coconut – this will toast very quickly in the hot pan so take care not to let it burn.
- Put all the toasted spices in a pestle and mortar and pound together. Add the grated ginger and garlic and grind together. Add the oil, ground almonds, salt and the rest of the spices and pound to make a dark oily paste.
- For the curry sauce, heat the spray oil gently in a non-stick saucepan. Add the onion and chillies and fry slowly until the onion is translucent, about 5–10 minutes. Add the spice paste to the pan and cook for a further 2 minutes, stirring constantly.
- Add the yogurt to the pan a spoonful at a time, stirring with each addition. Once the yogurt is added, pour in the tomatoes, stir and simmer gently for 20 minutes.

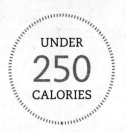

UNDER
250
CALORIES

Pear and walnut salad

240 calories

A very simple salad, but the flavours marry together beautifully. You can use other blue cheese if you like.

Serves 1   Preparation time: 5 minutes

½ tsp walnut oil (14 cals)
1 tbsp cider vinegar (4 cals)
salt and freshly ground black pepper
1 small dessert pear (48 cals)
80g (3¼oz) herb salad (11 cals)
25g (1oz) Roquefort cheese or other blue cheese (94 cals)
10g (⅓oz) walnut pieces (69 cals)

- Mix the walnut oil, vinegar and a little salt and pepper together to make a dressing.
- Cut the pear into quarters, remove the cores and cut each quarter into 4 slices.
- Arrange the herb salad on a serving plate and arrange the pear attractively over it. Crumble the cheese over the top, followed by the walnuts. Pour over the dressing and eat straight away.

My favourite mushroom curry

202 calories

Serves 2   Preparation time: 35 minutes   Cook time: 40 minutes

See main recipe on pages 131–2.

Additional ingredients:

250g (9oz) mushrooms (32 cals)

- Prepare the curry sauce according to pages 131–2.
- Slice the mushrooms and simply add to the curry sauce and simmer for 10 minutes. Serve.

Tarragon chicken

210 calories

This recipe uses chicken that is already cooked, so it can be put together in a few minutes – no cooking required.

Serves 1   Preparation time: 5 minutes

125g (4oz) roasted cooked chicken breast, skin removed (178 cals)

about 2 tbsp extra-light mayonnaise (30 cals)

1 tsp chopped fresh tarragon (2 cals)

salt and freshly ground black pepper

- Thinly slice the chicken and arrange on a plate.
- Mix the mayonnaise, tarragon and salt and pepper to taste together in a bowl. Dollop the herby mayonnaise over the chicken or serve in a pot on the side. Serve on a bed of lettuce leaves or as part of a salad, if you like.

Chicken satay

244 calories

This chicken satay can be either barbecued or grilled (broiled). They taste delicious served on a bed of spinach with some lime juice squeezed over – add on the appropriate calories if you are on a fast day. If using wooden skewers, make sure they are soaked in a bowl of water for at least 30 minutes before using to prevent them burning during cooking.

Serves 2   Preparation time: 10 minutes, plus 3–4 hours marinating
Cook time: 10 minutes

1 shallot, peeled and diced (5 cals)
1 garlic clove, peeled and crushed (3 cals)
2 tsp curry powder
1 level tbsp peanut butter (182 cals)
1 tsp runny honey (23 cals)
2 tbsp soy sauce (9 cals)
250g (9oz) skinless, boneless chicken breast, cut into cubes, about 2.5cm (1in) square (265 cals)

- To make the marinade, mix the shallot, garlic, curry powder, peanut butter, honey and soy sauce together in a bowl. Add the chicken and toss until the chicken is coated all over in the marinade. Leave to marinate in the refrigerator for 3–4 hours.
- Preheat the grill (broiler) to medium or light the barbecue. Thread the chicken cubes onto 2–4 skewers, leaving room between the chicken pieces to allow them to cook thoroughly. Grill (broil) for about 10 minutes, turning regularly, until cooked through. Serve immediately.

Posh chicken Kiev

224 calories

These chicken breasts are stuffed with garlicky cream cheese and wrapped in Parma ham (prosciutto). Serve on a bed of salad leaves (greens).

Serves 2   Preparation time: 10 minutes   Cook time: 25 minutes

½ tsp olive oil (14 cals)

1 garlic clove, peeled and very finely chopped (3 cals)

2 tbsp extra-light cream cheese (59 cals)

2 x 150g (5oz) skinless, boneless chicken breasts (318 cals)

2 slices Parma ham (prosciutto) (54 cals)

- Preheat the oven to 200°C/fan 180°C/400°F/Gas mark 6.
- Heat the olive oil in a small frying pan (skillet) and gently fry the garlic for 1–2 minutes until starting to brown. Remove from the heat and stir in the cream cheese.
- Prepare the chicken by making a slit down one side of the chicken breast to make a pocket, then fill each pocket equally with the garlicky cream cheese mixture. (This can get messy!) Wrap each chicken breast with a slice of Parma ham (prosciutto) and put onto a baking sheet (cookie sheet). Cook in the oven for 20–25 minutes or until the chicken is thoroughly cooked. Serve immediately.

Simple jerk chicken

211 calories

When marinating meat, fish or vegetables, cover the dish or bowl with cling film (plastic wrap) before placing it in the refrigerator to avoid cross-contamination.

Serves 1   Preparation time: 5 minutes, plus 30 minutes standing
Cook time: 30 minutes

1 tsp jerk seasoning mix
1 tsp roughly chopped fresh coriander (cilantro)
1 tsp olive oil (27 cals)
juice of ½ lemon (2 cals)
1 tsp honey (23 cals)
salt and freshly ground black pepper
1 × 150g (5oz) skinless, boneless chicken breast (159 cals)

- Mix the jerk seasoning, coriander (cilantro), olive oil, lemon juice, honey and a little salt and pepper together in a small bowl.
- Score the chicken and place in a small baking dish. Pour over the marinade and rub it all over the chicken. Leave to marinate in the refrigerator for at least 30 minutes.
- Preheat the oven to 220°C/fan 200°C/425°F/Gas mark 7.
- Cook the chicken in the oven for 20–30 minutes, or until cooked through. Serve.

Chicken with ginger and mango sauce

234 calories

Chicken and mango go so well together, and combined with fresh herbs and ginger, this dish will become a firm favourite.

Serves 2   Preparation time: 5 minutes   Cook time: 20 minutes

2 × 150g (5oz) skinless, boneless chicken breasts,
cut in half lengthways (318 cals)

½ tsp chopped fresh rosemary

½ tsp chopped fresh thyme

salt and freshly ground black pepper

1 tsp olive oil (27 cals)

100g (3½oz) mango pieces, chopped into
small pieces (65 cals)

2 tsp brown sugar (36 cals)

1 tbsp red wine vinegar (2 cals)

1 tbsp dry sherry (14 cals)

1 small thumb fresh root ginger, peeled and
finely grated (5 cals)

- Rub the chicken breast pieces with the herbs and a little salt and pepper.
- Heat the olive oil in a large frying pan (skillet) over a medium heat. Add the chicken and fry until golden brown and cooked through, about 8–10 minutes on each side. Remove the chicken from the pan with a slotted spoon, cover and keep warm.
- Return the pan to a medium heat, add the mango and fry for 2 minutes, then add the sugar, vinegar, sherry and ginger, stir well and continue to fry for a further 2 minutes. Pour the mango sauce over the chicken to serve.

Sweet onion chicken

235 calories

This is a hot and spicy yet fresh chicken dish. If you don't like too much spice, then deseed the chillies before using. Remember not to rub your face and eyes when handling chillies and to wash your hands, the knife and chopping (cutting) board after chopping them.

Serves 2   Preparation time: 10 minutes   Cook time: about 20 minutes

2 tsp sunflower oil (54 cals)
1 medium onion, peeled and finely chopped (65 cals)
2 bird's eye (Thai) chillies, finely chopped (1 cal)
3 garlic cloves, peeled and grated (9 cals)
2.5cm (1in) piece fresh root ginger, peeled and grated (5 cals)
a pinch of salt
1 tomato, diced (14 cals)
2 x 150g (5oz) skinless, boneless chicken breasts, cut into cubes (318 cals)
½ tsp ground cumin
1 tsp coarsely ground black pepper
1 small handful of fresh coriander (cilantro), chopped (3 cals)

- Heat the oil in a wide frying pan (skillet) over a medium-high heat. When hot, add the onion, chillies, garlic, ginger and salt and stir-fry for 2 minutes before reducing the heat and cooking gently for a further 5 minutes.
- Increase the heat to medium, toss in the tomato and stir-fry for 2 minutes. Add the chicken, cumin and pepper and stir-fry for a further 5 minutes.
- Reduce the heat to low, pour in 150ml (⅔ cup) water, stir and cook for another 5 minutes. If there seems to be too much liquid, increase the heat and boil for 1–2 minutes. Stir in the coriander (cilantro) before serving.

Quick turkey Bolognese

211 calories

Using turkey instead of the classic beef makes this lighter and healthier.

Serves 2   Preparation time: 5 minutes   Cook time: 25 minutes

1 tsp olive oil (27 cals)
1 small onion, peeled and chopped (22 cals)
½ green (bell) pepper, deseeded and diced (12 cals)
1 garlic clove, peeled (3 cals)
250g (9oz) turkey mince (ground turkey) (262 cals)
2 tbsp tomato purée (paste) (61 cals)
¼ chicken stock cube (9 cals)
½ tsp dried mixed herbs
½ tsp Worcestershire sauce (2 cals)
1 tbsp tomato ketchup (23 cals)

- Heat the olive oil in a medium-sized frying pan (skillet). Add the onion and green (bell) pepper and fry for 5 minutes before stirring in the garlic and frying for a further 2 minutes.
- Add the turkey mince (ground turkey) and cook, stirring regularly, until lightly browned. Stir in the tomato purée (paste), 150ml (⅔ cup) water, the stock cube, mixed herbs, Worcestershire sauce and tomato ketchup and simmer gently for 15 minutes before serving.

Slow-cooked chilli beef stew

206 calories

Similar to a classic chilli con carne, this stew is made with chunks of beef rather than mince (ground beef), giving it a distinctive flavour.

continued

Serves 6   Preparation time: 15 minutes   Cook time: about 1 hour

2 tsp sunflower oil (54 cals)

....

1 large onion, peeled and chopped (90 cals)

....

2 fresh green or red chillies, deseeded and

chopped into rings (3 cals)

....

3 garlic cloves, peeled and roughly chopped (9 cals)

....

600g (1¼lb) extra-lean casserole beef steak, diced (774 cals)

....

1 tsp mild chilli powder

....

1 tsp ground cumin

....

2 tsp paprika (14 cals)

....

1 tsp salt

....

1 tsp cocoa powder (unsweetened cocoa) (6 cals)

....

juice of 1 lime (3 cals)

....

1 × 400g (14oz) can chopped tomatoes (64 cals)

....

1 × 400g (14oz) can red kidney beans, drained

and rinsed (210 cals)

....

- Heat the oil in a large casserole over a medium heat, add the onion and gently fry for about 5 minutes. Add the chillies and garlic and fry for a further 2 minutes.
- Using a slotted spoon, remove the onion, chillies and garlic from the pan and turn the heat to high. Add the beef to the pan in 2 batches and fry until browned on all sides.
- Reduce the heat, return all the meat to the pan, together with the onion mixture and stir in the chilli powder, cumin, paprika, salt and cocoa. Finally, add the lime juice, canned tomatoes and kidney beans and stir well. Bring to the boil, reduce the heat and simmer gently for 30–40 minutes, stirring occasionally.
- Alternatively, transfer to a slow cooker and cook on low for about 8 hours or cook in a lidded casserole in an oven preheated to 160°C/fan 140°C/325°F/Gas mark 3 for 2 hours.

Chorizo and chickpea stew

204 calories

This chorizo stew serves four and freezes really well, so make a batch and freeze in individual portions, ready for other fast days.

Serves 4   Preparation time: 10 minutes   Cook time: about 30 minutes

1 tsp olive oil (27 cals)

1 large onion, peeled and diced (90 cals)

1 garlic clove, peeled and finely diced (3 cals)

1 green (bell) pepper, deseeded and diced (24 cals)

80g (3¼oz) chorizo, diced (233 cals)

1 × 400g (14oz) can chopped tomatoes (64 cals)

500ml (generous 2 cups) vegetable stock, fresh or made with 1 stock cube (35 cals)

1 × 400g (14oz) can chickpeas, drained and rinsed (276 cals)

½ tsp chilli flakes (red pepper flakes) (optional)

2 tbsp tomato purée (paste) (61 cals)

1 small handful of fresh parsley, roughly chopped (3 cals)

- Heat the olive oil in a wide saucepan, add the onion, garlic and green (bell) pepper and gently fry for 8 minutes. Increase the heat to high, add the diced chorizo and stir-fry for 2 minutes until the chorizo has a golden tinge and the oil has run out.
- Reduce the heat to low, add the canned tomatoes, vegetable stock, chickpeas, chilli flakes (red pepper flakes) and tomato purée (paste) and simmer gently for 20 minutes. Sprinkle the chopped parsley over the top and serve.

Sizzling pork boats

230 calories

This is a fun and tasty dish, inspired by trips to my favourite Mexican restaurant.

Serves 1   Preparation time: 8 minutes, plus 5 minutes standing
Cook time: about 8 minutes

1 lean pork steak (100g/3½oz trimmed weight) (147 cals)
½ tsp paprika (3 cals)
½ tsp mild chilli powder
½ tsp ground cumin
a pinch of salt
½ tsp soft brown sugar (11 cals)
1 tsp sunflower oil (27 cals)
½ green (bell) pepper, deseeded and cut into thin strips (12 cals)
½ red (bell) pepper, deseeded and cut into thin strips (26 cals)
4 little gem lettuce leaves (4 cals)

- Cut any fat off the pork then cut into thin strips – you want the slices to be similar in length and size to the sliced peppers.
- Mix the spices, salt, sugar, oil and 2 tablespoons water together in a bowl. Place the pork and peppers in the bowl and toss thoroughly. Leave to stand for 5 minutes to allow the flavours to infuse.
- Heat a wide flat frying pan (skillet) over a medium heat and add the pork, peppers and any juices into the pan. It will sizzle as you start to cook and continue to sizzle gently through cooking. Stir-fry for 6–8 minutes or until the pork is cooked through.
- Place the lettuce leaves on a serving plate and scoop the pork filling into them equally. Serve while piping hot.

Fresh tuna goujons with pineapple salsa

238 calories

The bold flavours of the pineapple salsa complement the tuna in this dish.

Serves 2   Preparation time: 10 minutes   Cook time: 5 minutes

1 × 225g (8oz) can pineapple chunks in juice,
drained and chopped into small chunks (106 cals)

¼ tsp chilli flakes (red pepper flakes)

1 small handful of fresh coriander (cilantro),
finely chopped (3 cals)

1 tsp lemon juice

2 × 200g (7oz) fresh tuna steaks (272 cals)

1 level tbsp plain (all-purpose) flour, seasoned with salt
and freshly ground black pepper (68 cals)

1 tsp olive oil (27 cals)

- Combine the chopped pineapple, chilli flakes (red pepper flakes), coriander (cilantro) and lemon juice in a small bowl and set aside while you prepare the tuna.
- Cut each tuna steak into 4 strips and toss in the seasoned flour until just coated.
- Heat the olive oil in a frying pan (skillet) over a high heat. The oil needs to be glimmering hot before adding the tuna. Fry the tuna for just 1–2 minutes, turning once.
- Pile the salsa onto 2 serving plates, arrange the tuna strips on top and serve.

Spanish fish stew

243 calories

Full of colour and flavour, this one-pot dish is ideal to eat when fasting.

Serves 2   Preparation time: 10 minutes   Cook time: 35 minutes

1 tsp olive oil (27 cals)

½ onion, peeled and finely chopped (27 cals)

1 garlic clove, peeled and finely chopped (3 cals)

½ celery stick, finely chopped (2 cals)

½ green (bell) pepper, deseeded and diced (12 cals)

½ yellow (bell) pepper, deseeded and diced (21 cals)

1 medium tomato, chopped (14 cals)

5 tbsp white wine (56 cals)

¼ tsp cayenne pepper (3 cals)

½ tsp paprika (3 cals)

400ml (1¾ cups) fish stock, fresh or made from
1 stock cube (35 cals)

100g (3½oz) new potatoes (2–3 depending on size),
halved (70 cals)

1 skinless cod fillet, about 130g (4½oz),
cut into chunks (104 cals)

100g (3½oz) raw king prawns (king shrimp)
(76 cals)

50g (1¼oz)) frozen peas (34 cals)

juice of ½ lemon (2 cals)

1 tsp chopped fresh parsley

freshly ground black pepper

continued

- Heat the oil in a large saucepan over a low heat. Add the onion, garlic, celery and (bell) peppers and fry gently for about 5 minutes until softened. Add the tomato and cook for a further 1 minute.
- Increase the heat to medium, add the wine and let it simmer vigorously for about 4 minutes. Stir in the spices and stock and bring to the boil. Add the potatoes and cook for 15 minutes.
- Add the fish, prawns (shrimps) and peas to the pan, then reduce the heat, cover and simmer for 6–8 minutes, or until the fish is just cooked. Stir in the lemon juice and parsley and season to taste with pepper.

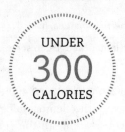

UNDER

300

CALORIES

Falafel and butternut squash salad

299 calories

It's very easy to make your own falafels and these ones are extremely healthy as they are baked in the oven.

Serves 2   Preparation time: 10 minutes   Cook time: about 20 minutes

1 × 400g (14oz) can chickpeas, rinsed and drained (304 cals)

2 garlic cloves, peeled (6 cals)

juice of ½ lemon (2 cals)

a few fresh coriander (cilantro) leaves (optional)

1 tsp cornflour (cornstarch) (28 cals)

1 tsp ground cumin

½ tsp ground coriander

½ tsp cayenne pepper (3 cals)

a pinch of salt

1 tsp olive oil (27 cals)

1 × 450g (1lb) butternut squash, deseeded, peeled and sliced into fingers (162 cals)

salt and freshly ground black pepper

1 romaine lettuce heart, leaves roughly torn (20 cals)

continued

20 cherry tomatoes, halved (45 cals)

lemon wedges, to serve

- Preheat the oven to 200°C/fan 180°C/400°F/Gas mark 6.
- Place the chickpeas, garlic, lemon juice, coriander (cilantro) leaves, cornflour (cornstarch), all the spices and the salt in a food processor and pulse until finely chopped but not puréed. Divide the mixture into 6 portions, shape each portion into a ball, then flatten slightly with the palm of your hand.
- Brush the falafels with a little olive oil on both sides and arrange on a non-stick baking tray. Brush the butternut squash fingers with the remaining olive oil, or use a little 1 cal spray and put the butternut squash on the baking tray as well. Season with a little salt and pepper and cook in the oven for about 20 minutes or until the falafel are brown and the butternut squash is cooked.
- Arrange the lettuce and tomatoes on 2 serving plates, scatter on the butternut squash fingers and place 3 falafels on each plate. Serve with 1 or 2 lemon wedges on the side.

Puy lentils and feta cheese salad

272 calories

This filling salad is so tasty. You can also use ready-to-eat lentils to make this salad super quick, if you like.

Serves 1   Preparation time: 5 minutes   Cook time: 25 minutes

40g (1½oz) dried Puy lentils (119 cals)

15 cherry tomatoes (34 cals)

50g (1¾oz) baby spinach leaves (12 cals)

30g (1¼oz) pickled sweet peppers in brine, drained
and roughly chopped (33 cals)

2 fresh basil leaves, shredded

1 tbsp balsamic vinegar (14 cals)

salt and freshly ground black pepper

30g (1¼oz) light feta cheese (60 cals)

- Cook the Puy lentils in a pan of boiling water for about 25 minutes, or according to the packet instructions. Leave the lentils to cool slightly; they are perfect warm but not hot.
- When the lentils are warm, combine them with the cherry tomatoes, baby spinach, sweet peppers and basil leaves in a large bowl. Pour the balsamic vinegar over, season with a little salt and pepper and toss well.
- Transfer to a serving dish, crumble the feta over the top and serve while still warm.

Fresh tuna Niçoise

268 calories

Don't be surprised that there's no egg in this recipe. It's been sacrificed in favour of a whole tuna steak. If you want to add a large boiled egg, feel free – it's 89 calories.

Serves 1   Preparation time: 8 minutes   Cook time: 2 minutes

100g (3½oz) fresh tuna steak (136 cals)
salt and freshly ground black pepper
1 tsp extra-virgin olive oil (27 cals)
1 tsp white wine vinegar (1 cals)
a pinch of sugar (4 cals)
1 tsp capers (1 cals)
1 fresh basil leaf, shredded
1 little gem lettuce, separated into leaves (22 cals)
10 cherry tomatoes, halved (22 cals)
40g (1½oz) green beans, cooked from fresh or frozen (10 cals)
4 anchovy fillets (24 cals)
4 large black olives (21 cals)

- Place the tuna on a plate and rub all over with a little salt and pepper. Leave to rest for a few minutes while you make the rest of the salad.
- Mix the olive oil, vinegar, sugar, capers and basil leaf together in a small bowl and set aside.
- In a serving dish, arrange the lettuce leaves, tomatoes and green beans. Place the anchovies and black olives towards the outside of the plate and pour the dressing over.

- Heat a frying pan (skillet) over a high heat until the pan is very hot. Do not add the tuna until you are sure it is searing hot. Cook the tuna for 1 minute, then turn over and cook for 30 seconds. It needs to be charred on the outside but a little pink inside.
- Transfer the tuna to a chopping (cutting) board and cut into thin slices. Arrange the slices in the centre of the salad and eat while still warm.

Mushroom frittata
265 calories

A frittata is similar to an omelette, but is thicker and more substantial and laced with onions.

Serves 1   Preparation time: 2 minutes   Cook time: 20 minutes

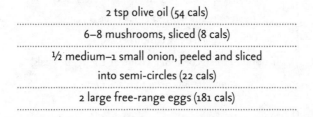

2 tsp olive oil (54 cals)
6–8 mushrooms, sliced (8 cals)
½ medium–1 small onion, peeled and sliced into semi-circles (22 cals)
2 large free-range eggs (181 cals)

- Heat 1 teaspoon of the olive oil in a small frying pan (skillet) over a medium heat. Add the mushrooms and cook for 4–5 minutes, then remove with a slotted spoon. Add the remaining oil and the onion to the pan and fry for 10 minutes, stirring regularly. Turn the heat down if the onion is browning or catching on the base of the pan. The onion should be cooked and starting to caramelize at this point.
- Crack the eggs into a bowl and whisk with a fork. Reduce the heat under the onion pan to low and arrange the onions relatively evenly over the base. Pour in the eggs, making sure that the base of the pan is covered. If you have a lid, place it on top at this point; if not, cover with a plate and cook for 3 minutes. Add the mushrooms, cover again and cook for a further 2 minutes. Serve immediately.

Oven-baked mushroom pilaf

294 calories

If you use quick-cook rice in this dish, then adjust the cooking time.

Serves 2   Preparation time: 10 minutes   Cook time: 1 hour

½ tbsp pine nuts (69 cals)
1 tsp olive oil (27 cals)
1 red onion, peeled and cut into thin wedges (54 cals)
1 tsp turmeric
250g (9oz) brown mushrooms, sliced (32 cals)
100g (3½oz) brown rice, rinsed (357 cals)
1 dessertspoon raisins (27 cals)
300ml (1¼ cups) chicken or vegetable stock, fresh or made with ½ stock cube (17 cals)
juice of ½ lemon (2 cals)
1 handful of fresh coriander (cilantro), chopped (3 cals)
salt and freshly ground black pepper

- Preheat the oven to 200°C/fan 180°C/400°F/Gas mark 6.
- Toast the pine nuts in a dry frying pan (skillet), then remove from the heat and set aside.
- Heat the olive oil in an ovenproof casserole, add the onion and turmeric and fry for 3 minutes. Add the mushrooms and fry for a further 2 minutes. Tip in the rice, raisins and stock and stir well. Bring to a gentle simmer, then cover with a lid and place in the oven. Cook for 45–55 minutes, checking if you need to add a little more water halfway through, until the rice is tender.
- Stir in the toasted pine nuts, lemon juice, coriander (cilantro) and a little salt and pepper to taste before serving.

Spinach and pea rice

298 calories

This spiced brown rice is so tasty it is a meal in its own right.

Serves 2   Preparation time: 10 minutes   Cook time: about 1 hour

100g (3½oz) brown rice, rinsed (357 cals)
1 tbsp sunflower oil (99 cals)
1 onion, peeled and chopped (54 cals)
1 bird's eye (Thai) chilli, deseeded and finely chopped (1 cals)
½ tsp aniseed seeds (optional)
½ tsp garam masala
½ tsp ground cumin
a pinch of salt
100g (3½oz) frozen spinach, defrosted (21 cals)
90g (3¼oz) frozen peas, about 2 big handfuls (59 cals)
1 handful of fresh coriander (cilantro), chopped (3 cals)
juice of ½ lemon (2 cals)

- Cook the brown rice in a pan of boiling water for about 35–40 minutes, or according to the packet instructions. Drain.
- Heat the oil in a wide frying pan (skillet) over a medium heat. Add the onion, chilli and aniseed (if using), then stir, reduce the heat and cook for 5–10 minutes until the onion is translucent.
- Add the ground spices and salt to the pan and stir for 30 seconds. Add the spinach and peas and increase the heat to medium. Stir-fry for 2–3 minutes, then add the cooked rice, coriander (cilantro) and lemon juice. Stir-fry for a further 2–3 minutes until everything is completely mixed and the rice is warm.

Red pepper and lentil bake

293 calories

This is an ideal recipe to make if you are feeding several people. It's also great reheated the next day in the microwave.

Serves 4   Preparation time: 10 minutes   Cook time: about 50 minutes

1 tsp olive oil (27 cals)

1 large onion, peeled and finely chopped (72 cals)

1 garlic clove, peeled and finely chopped (3 cals)

100g (3½oz) dried Puy lentils (297 cals)

1 vegetable stock cube (33 cals)

8 red (bell) peppers, deseeded and chopped (410 cals)

1 large cooking apple, peeled, cored and chopped (80 cals)

2 tsp dried basil (3 cals)

50ml (scant ¼ cup) white wine (33 cals)

1 × 400g (14oz) can chopped tomatoes (64 cals)

25g (1oz) mature (sharp) Cheddar cheese, grated (104 cals)

10g (⅓oz) Parmesan cheese, finely grated (45 cals)

- Preheat the oven to 180°C/fan 160°C/350°F/Gas mark 4.
- Heat the olive oil gently in a large saucepan, add the onion and garlic and fry for 5 minutes or until the onion turns translucent. Add the lentils, stir, then add 600ml (2½ cups) water and crumble in the stock cube. Bring to the boil, then reduce the heat and simmer for 25 minutes. Next, add the red (bell) peppers, apple, basil, white wine and canned tomatoes and mix well.
- Transfer the mixture to an ovenproof baking dish and sprinkle the 2 grated cheeses over the top. Cook in the oven for 30 minutes. Serve immediately or cool and freeze in individual portions.

My favourite vegetable curry

281 calories

Serves 2   Preparation time: 40 minutes   Cook time: 50 minutes

See main recipe on pages 131–2.

Additional ingredients:

1 medium carrot, peeled and chopped into
large chunks (35 cals)

....

100g (3½oz) swede (rutabaga), parsnip or celeriac
(celery root), peeled and chopped into chunks (24 cals)

....

1 small onion, peeled and cut into eighths
lengthways (36 cals)

....

1 tsp sunflower oil (27 cals)

....

100g (3½oz) cauliflower, cut into 6–8 small
florets (34 cals)

....

100g (3½oz) broccoli, cut into 6–8 florets (33 cals)

....

- Preheat the oven to 190°C/fan 170°C/375°F/Gas mark 5.
- Place the chopped carrot, swede (rutabaga) and onion on a baking tray. Add the oil and mix in thoroughly, then roast in the oven for 15 minutes.
- Prepare the curry sauce according to pages 131–2. Add the roasted vegetables, cauliflower and broccoli and stir into the sauce. Simmer gently for 15–20 minutes or until all the vegetables are tender. Serve.

My favourite chicken curry
300 calories

Serves 2   Preparation time: 35 minutes   Cook time: 45 minutes

See main recipe on pages 131–2.

Additional ingredients:
1 x 215g (7oz) skinless, boneless chicken breasts, chopped
into bite-sized pieces (228 cals)

....

- Follow the basic curry recipe on pages 131–2, then add the chicken pieces and simmer gently for 12–15 minutes or until cooked through. Serve.

Middle Eastern chicken
272 calories

This is my take on a chicken shawarma. The chicken needs to be marinated for eight hours or overnight, but then it's quick to cook and serve.

Serves 2   Preparation time: 10 minutes, plus 8 hours marinating
Cook time: about 10 minutes

2 × 150g (5oz) skinless, boneless chicken breasts,
thinly sliced (318 cals)

....

1 tsp sunflower oil (27 cals)

....

For the marinade:

2 level tbsp low-fat plain yogurt (17 cals)

....

1 garlic clove, peeled and crushed (3 cals)

....

salt and freshly ground black pepper

1 cardamom pod

½ tsp allspice

juice of ½ lemon (2 cals)

For the sauce:

1 level tsp tahini (sesame seed paste) (91 cals)

½ garlic clove, peeled and crushed (2 cals)

juice of 1 lemon (2 cals)

1 level tbsp low-fat plain yogurt (8 cals)

For the salad:

½ iceberg lettuce (200g/7oz), shredded (26 cals)

2 spring onions (scallions), trimmed and shredded (9 cals)

2 medium tomatoes, thinly sliced (29 cals)

100g (3½oz) cucumber, peeled and thinly sliced (10 cals)

- Mix all the marinade ingredients together in a large shallow bowl and add the chicken strips. Turn the chicken until it is well coated in the marinade, then cover and chill in the refrigerator for 8 hours, or overnight.
- When you are ready to cook the chicken, make the sauce by simply combining all the sauce ingredients in a small bowl and stirring well.
- Heat the oil in a wok or wide frying pan (skillet) over a medium-high heat. When it's sizzling hot, toss in the chicken, including any marinade, and stir-fry for 6–8 minutes or until cooked through.
- Pile the salad ingredients onto 2 serving plates and arrange the chicken on top. Serve the sauce separately or drizzled over.

Chilli chicken salad

274 calories

This chicken is marinated for an hour to make it beautifully tender when cooked.

Serves 1   Preparation time: 10 minutes, plus 1 hour marinating
Cook time: 10 minutes

2 spring onions (scallions), trimmed and
finely chopped (9 cals)

2 garlic cloves, peeled and finely chopped (6 cals)

juice of 1 lemon (4 cals)

½ tsp honey (47 cals)

½ tsp paprika (3 cals)

¼ tsp mild chilli powder

salt and freshly ground black pepper

1 × 150g (5oz) chicken breast fillet, cut into 8 pieces (159 cals)

For the salad:

¼ iceberg lettuce, shredded (14 cals)

100g (3½oz) cucumber (5cm/2in piece), diced (10 cals)

2 vine-ripened tomatoes, diced (20 cals)

juice of ½ lemon (2 cals)

- First, make a marinade by combining the spring onions (scallions), garlic, lemon juice, honey, spices and a little salt and pepper in a bowl. Add the chicken pieces to the bowl, making sure that they are fully coated in the marinade. Cover and leave to marinate in the refrigerator for about 1 hour.
- When you are ready to cook the chicken, preheat the grill (broiler) to medium. Place the chicken pieces on the grill pan

and grill (broil) for 8–10 minutes, turning once. They should be brown and crispy all over and the chicken cooked through.

- Place the lettuce, cucumber and tomatoes in a serving bowl and arrange the still-warm chicken over the top. Mix the lemon juice with salt and pepper to taste to make a dressing and pour over the top. Serve immediately.

Mediterranean chicken with feta
259 calories

This is a tasty and summery chicken dish.

Serves 2   Preparation time: 5 minutes   Cook time: 45 minutes

2 x 150g (5oz) skinless, boneless chicken breasts (318 cals)

1 tbsp tomato purée (paste) (30 cals)

1 tsp chopped fresh basil

1 tsp olive oil (27 cals)

1 garlic clove, peeled and finely sliced (3 cals)

1 x 400g (14oz) can whole tomatoes (64 cals)

a pinch of salt

1 tbsp red wine vinegar (1 cal)

25g (1oz) light feta cheese, cut into small cubes (75 cals)

- Cut each chicken breast into 2 pieces and lightly score on both sides. Rub the tomato purée (paste) and half the basil over the 4 pieces of chicken and leave to rest while you prepare the sauce.
- Heat the olive oil gently in a non-stick saucepan, add the garlic and fry for 1–2 minutes until just starting to brown. Add the canned tomatoes, salt and the remaining basil and simmer over a medium heat for 10 minutes. Reduce the heat and break up the tomatoes with the back of a wooden spoon. Add the red wine

continued

vinegar and continue to simmer gently for another 10 minutes.

- Meanwhile, preheat the grill (broiler) to medium. Arrange the chicken pieces on the grill pan and grill (broil) for 7–8 minutes on each side. The chicken should be cooked through and turning golden all over.
- Add the chicken and feta to the tomato sauce and stir in. Heat for a further 2–3 minutes, then serve.

Grilled chicken topped with sun-dried tomatoes and olives

293 calories

If you can't find rocket (arugula) salad try a mixed leaf salad instead.

Serves 1   Preparation time: 2 minutes   Cook time: 16 minutes

1 x 150g (5oz) skinless, boneless chicken breast (159 cals)

4 (about 10g/⅓oz) sun-dried tomato pieces in oil (50 cals)

5 large black olives, stoned (pitted) (26 cals)

1 small bag (80g/3¼oz) rocket (arugula) salad (58 cals)

- Preheat the grill (broiler) to medium-high.
- Cut the chicken into 2 pieces and lightly score it on both sides. Place in a bowl. Roughly chop the tomato and black olives and add to the bowl. Press the mixture into the scores on the chicken and rub any remaining bits over the top.
- Put the chicken on the grill pan and grill (broil) for 7–8 minutes on each side. Check that the chicken is cooked all the way through.
- Arrange the rocket (arugula) salad on a serving plate, put the chicken on top and serve.

Harissa roasted chicken, shallots and sweet potato

261 calories

This is a great combination of flavours and is very simple to put together.

Serves 1   Preparation time: 5 minutes, plus 30 minutes marinating
Cook time: about 25 minutes

1 x 150g (5oz) skinless, boneless chicken breast (159 cals)

½ small sweet potato (75g/3oz), peeled and
chopped roughly into large cubes (65 cals)

2 shallots, peeled and quartered (24 cals)

1 tbsp harissa paste (13 cals)

- Cut the chicken breast into 3 or 4 pieces and place in a bowl with the sweet potato and shallots.
- In a small bowl, combine the harissa paste with 1 tablespoon water. Pour over the chicken and vegetables and mix thoroughly, making sure everything is coated. Cover and leave to marinate for about 30 minutes.
- Preheat the oven to 220°C/fan 200°C/425°F/Gas mark 7.
- Transfer the chicken and vegetables to a wide baking dish and cook in the oven for 18–25 minutes. Check that the chicken is cooked through before serving.
- This dish works equally well with a green vegetable such as wilted spinach or steamed broccoli, or with a light salad.

Homemade burgers

267 calories

Serve these healthy burgers with a fresh green salad, adding on the appropriate calories if you are on a fast day.

Serves 2   Preparation time: 5 minutes, plus 1 hour chilling
Cook time: 8–10 minutes

250g (9oz) extra-lean minced (ground) beef (435 cals)

1 shallot, peeled and finely diced (5 cals)

1 small garlic clove, peeled and finely chopped (3 cals)

½ tsp dried herbs or 1 tsp chopped fresh basil,
parsley or coriander (cilantro)

1 tsp Worcestershire sauce (3 cals)

1 small free-range egg, beaten (60 cals)

salt and freshly ground black pepper

1 tsp olive oil (27 cals)

- Place all the ingredients except the olive oil in a large bowl and mix together by hand until fully combined. Divide the mixture into 4 equal pieces and roll each one into a ball, then flatten with the palm of your hand to make a burger shape. Place the burgers on a plate, cover and chill in the refrigerator for about an hour.
- Heat the olive oil in a wide frying pan (skillet) and fry for 8–10 minutes, turning once. Serve immediately.

Peppered beef with mustard sauce

296 calories

If you use extra-lean beef you can eat red meat on a fast day. Serve with a simple green salad.

Serves 1   Preparation time: 10 minutes, plus 5–60 minutes standing
Cook time: 15 minutes, plus 5 minutes resting

½ tsp olive oil (14 cals)

150g (5oz) extra-lean beef escalope (scallop) (184 cals)

1 tsp roughly ground black pepper

a pinch of salt

For the mustard sauce:

½ tsp olive oil (14 cals)

½ shallot, peeled and very finely diced (3 cals)

1 tbsp brandy (31 cals)

½ tsp English mustard (3 cals)

1 tsp Dijon mustard (7 cals)

1 tbsp light crème fraîche (40 cals)

- Rub a little olive oil over both sides of the steak. Sprinkle the roughly ground pepper on a plate with the salt, add the steak and turn until it is coated on all sides with the pepper. Leave to rest for at least 5 minutes or up to an hour at room temperature.
- Heat a frying pan (skillet) over a very high heat. When the pan is properly hot, add the peppered steak and cook for 2–4 minutes on each side, depending on thickness and how you like your steak cooked. Don't overcook as the meat will become tough. When cooked, cover and leave to rest for 5 minutes while you finish the mustard sauce.
- To make the sauce, heat the olive oil in a small frying pan over

continued

a low heat and toss in the diced shallot. Cook gently for 5–10 minutes until translucent. Increase the heat to medium, add the brandy and let it bubble for 1 minute before reducing the heat again. Add both mustards and the crème fraîche, stir well and cook for a further 2 minutes.

- Place the steak on a serving plate and pour the sauce over to serve.

Shanghai-style pork
299 calories

A normal tenderloin is around 400g (14oz), so you should be able to buy a whole one and use half. This is delicious served with pak choi.

Serves 2   Preparation time: 10 minutes   Cook time: about 35 minutes, plus 5 minutes resting

190g (7oz) pork tenderloin fillet (467 cals)
1 green (bell) pepper, deseeded and cut into strips (24 cals)
1 tbsp dark soy sauce (4 cals)
1 tbsp mirin (rice wine) or dry sherry (35 cals)
1 tsp sesame oil (27 cals)
1 tsp runny honey (23 cals)
1 garlic clove, peeled and crushed or grated (3 cals)
1 thumb fresh root ginger, peeled and grated (5 cals)
100ml (scant ½ cup) chicken stock, fresh or made with ¼ stock cube (9 cals)

- Preheat the oven to 200°C/fan 180°C/400°F/Gas mark 6.
- Place the pork in a small ovenproof dish and scatter the green (bell) pepper around it.
- In a small bowl, mix the soy sauce, mirin (rice wine), oil, honey, garlic, ginger and chicken stock. Pour the sauce over the pork and cook in the oven for 25 minutes, basting with the sauce occasionally. *continued*

- Remove the sauce and peppers from the dish and keep them warm. Put the pork back into the oven and roast for a further 10–15 minutes, then leave in the baking dish to rest for a further 5 minutes. Slice and serve with the sauce.

Sweet and sour pork
298 calories

A classic Chinese takeaway (takeout) favourite, this dish is very easy to make.

Serves 2   Preparation time: 10 minutes   Cook time: 14 minutes

1 × 175g (6oz) lean pork tenderloin fillet,
thinly sliced (394 cals)

½ level tbsp plain (all-purpose) flour, seasoned with
salt and freshly ground black pepper (34 cals)

2 tsp olive oil (54 cals)

1 garlic clove, peeled and finely chopped (3 cals)

4 spring onions (scallions), trimmed and shredded (18 cals)

½ red (bell) pepper, deseeded and finely sliced (26 cals)

½ yellow (bell) pepper, deseeded and finely sliced (21 cals)

1 level tsp granulated sugar (16 cals)

1 tbsp white wine vinegar (3 cals)

1 tsp tomato purée (paste) (8 cals)

1 tbsp light soy sauce (4 cals)

1 tbsp dry sherry (14 cals)

- Toss the pork in the seasoned flour until lightly coated.
- Heat the olive oil in a wide saucepan or wok over a medium-high heat. Add the pork and stir-fry until just cooked, about 4–5 minutes. Remove the pork from the pan with a slotted spoon, cover and keep warm.

continued

- Return the pan to a medium heat, add the garlic and spring onions (scallions) and stir-fry for 1 minute before adding the (bell) peppers and stir-frying for a further 3 minutes.
- Return the pork to the pan and stir in the sugar, vinegar, tomato purée (paste), soy sauce, 50ml (scant ¼ cup) water and the sherry. Simmer for 3 more minutes before serving.

Pork stir-fry with water chestnuts
289 calories

The addition of water chestnuts in this stir-fry brings a crunch to the tender pork and vegetables.

Serves 2 Preparation time: 5 minutes Cook time: 10 minutes

1 tsp sunflower oil (27 cals)

½ onion, peeled and finely chopped (32 cals)

½ red (bell) pepper, deseeded and cut into strips (26 cals)

160g (5½oz) lean pork tenderloin, cut into
thin strips (394 cals)

1 red chilli, deseeded and cut into rings (3 cals)

1 garlic clove, peeled and finely chopped (3 cals)

1 × 225g (8oz) can water chestnuts, drained
and sliced (70 cals)

1 tbsp dark soy sauce (4 cals)

½ tbsp mirin (rice wine) or sherry (18 cals)

- Heat the oil in a wok or wide saucepan over a medium-high heat, add the onion and red (bell) pepper and stir-fry for 3 minutes. Add the pork, chilli and garlic and stir-fry for a further 3 minutes. Add the water chestnuts and cook for 2 minutes.
- Blend the soy sauce and mirin (rice wine) or sherry together in a small bowl, then mix into the stir-fry. Cook for a further 2 minutes, then serve.

Roasted pork with plums

273 calories

The plums and pork are roasted separately in the oven here. If you don't have an ovenproof frying pan (skillet) then transfer the browned pork to a roasting pan before cooking in the oven.

Serves 2   Preparation time: 10 minutes   Cook time: 30 minutes, plus 10 minutes resting

175g (6oz) pork tenderloin fillet (430 cals)
1 tsp olive oil (27 cals)
salt and freshly ground black pepper
3 fresh plums, pitted and cut into quarters (60 cals)
2 fresh rosemary sprigs
¼ vanilla pod (bean), split
1 level tsp granulated sugar (16 cals)
1 tbsp balsamic vinegar (12 cals)

- Preheat the oven to 210°C/fan 190°C/410°F/Gas mark 6½.
- Rub the pork all over with the olive oil and a little salt and pepper. Heat an ovenproof frying pan (skillet) over a high heat. When the pan is hot, flash-fry the pork for 2 minutes on each side until brown.
- Transfer the pork to the oven and cook for 10–15 minutes or until cooked through. Remove from the oven, cover with foil and rest for 10 minutes before serving.
- Meanwhile, place the plums on a baking tray, add the rosemary and vanilla pod (bean), then sprinkle with the sugar and drizzle over the balsamic vinegar. Cook the plums at the top of the oven for 20–25 minutes until tender and beginning to break down. Remove from the oven and discard the rosemary and vanilla pod.
- Put the pork onto a chopping (cutting) board and cut into thin slices. Arrange the pork on 2 serving plates and serve with the roasted plums.

Maple-glazed pork

298 calories

A simple, tangy glaze of maple syrup, vinegar and mustard really enhances the flavour of the meat in this dish.

Serves 2   Preparation time: 5 minutes   Cook time: 30–40 minutes,
plus 10 minutes resting

1 level tsp butter (watch out – this isn't a lot!) (34 cals)
200g (7oz) pork tenderloin fillet (492 cals)
½ tsp dried sage
salt and freshly ground black pepper
1 tbsp maple syrup (53 cals)
1 tbsp apple cider vinegar (2 cals)
2 tsp Dijon mustard (14 cals)

- Preheat the oven to 200°C/fan 180°C/400°F/Gas mark 6.
- Rub the butter all over the pork and sprinkle with sage and a little salt and pepper. Place the pork in a small ovenproof dish and roast in the oven for 30–40 minutes, depending on size. Check the pork after 30 minutes. If it's cooked it should look pleasingly brown and be cooked all the way through. Remove from the oven, cover and leave to rest for 10 minutes.
- Meanwhile, drain any juices and browned bits from the baking dish into a small saucepan, add the maple syrup, vinegar and mustard and heat gently on the hob for 2 minutes.
- Spread a little of the glaze over the meat, then transfer the pork to a chopping (cutting) board and cut into 1cm (½in) slices. Arrange the pork on serving plates and pour the rest of the glaze over the top.

Pork and apricot skewers

286 calories

The sweet apricots make for a delicious taste combination with the salty pork. Serve with a green vegetable such as mangetout (snow peas) or purple sprouting broccoli. If using wooden skewers, make sure they are soaked in a bowl of water for at least 30 minutes before using to prevent them burning during cooking.

Serves 1   Preparation time: 5 minutes, plus 15 minutes soaking
Cook time: 16 minutes, plus 2 minutes resting

4 dried apricots (38 cals)
a pinch of salt
90g (3¼oz) lean pork tenderloin, cut into 6 chunks (221 cals)
1 tsp olive oil (27 cals)

- Place the apricots in a small bowl and cover with boiling water. Make sure that the apricots are just covered with the water. Leave to soak for 15 minutes until soft.
- Sprinkle the salt over the pork chunks and rub the salt into the meat.
- Preheat the grill (broiler) to medium.
- Thread the pork and apricots alternately onto skewers. You should make 2 skewers with 3 pieces of pork and 2 apricots apiece, leaving room between the pork and apricots to allow them to cook thoroughly. Brush the skewers all over with the olive oil and place on the grill pan. Grill (broil) for 7–8 minutes on each side. Check that the pork is cooked through and browned all over. Leave to rest for 2 minutes before serving.

Caribbean-style pork

299 calories

Be sure to buy light coconut milk for this delicious dish.

Serves 4   Preparation time: 10 minutes   Cook time: 30 minutes

½ tsp sunflower oil (14 cals)

275g (10oz) lean pork tenderloin, trimmed and
cut into strips (676 cals)

1 red onion, peeled and cut into wedges (54 cals)

½ tbsp jerk paste (20 cals)

½ yellow (bell) pepper, deseeded and sliced (21 cals)

1 green (bell) pepper, deseeded and sliced (24 cals)

1 small carrot, peeled and cut into ribbons using a
vegetable peeler (28 cals)

½ x 400ml (14fl oz) can light coconut milk (146 cals)

1 x 400g (14oz) can chopped tomatoes (64 cals)

1 x 210g (7oz) can red kidney beans,
rinsed and drained (120 cals)

100g (3½oz) baby leaf spinach (25 cals)

1 handful of fresh flat-leaf (Italian) parsley, roughly
chopped (3 cals)

- Heat the oil in a large wok or frying pan (skillet) over a medium heat. Add the pork strips and fry for 8–10 minutes, stirring frequently, until browned and cooked through. Remove from the pan with a slotted spoon, cover and keep warm.
- Reduce the heat in the pan slightly, add the onion and cook for 5 minutes before adding the jerk paste, (bell) peppers and carrot. Cook for a further 5 minutes.

- Stir in the coconut milk and chopped tomatoes and cook for 5 minutes, then add the kidney beans and pork and cook for another 5 minutes. Add the spinach, stir through and cook for 1 more minute. Sprinkle with the parsley and serve.

Ham and lentil stew
256 calories

This healthy stew serves four, so divide it into individual portions and freeze for other days.

Serves 4 Preparation time: 5 minutes Cook time: 1¼ hours

1 tsp olive oil (27 cals)
1 large onion, peeled and diced (86 cals)
2 medium carrots, peeled and diced (70 cals)
50g (1¾oz) pearl barley, rinsed (180 cals)
1 litre (4 cups) chicken stock, fresh or made with 2 stock cubes (70 cals)
50g (1¾oz) Puy lentils, rinsed (148 cals)
1 medium potato, peeled and chopped into small dice (169 calories)
250g (9oz) cooked ham, shredded (268 cals)
1 small handful of fresh parsley, roughly chopped (3 cals)

- Heat the olive oil in a wide saucepan or casserole over a low heat. Add the onion and carrots and fry very gently for 10 minutes until the onion is translucent. Stir the pearl barley into the pan and pour in the stock. Bring to the boil, then reduce the heat and simmer for 40 minutes.
- Add the lentils and diced potato, top up with 1 litre (4 cups) water and cook for a further 30 minutes.
- Add the shredded ham to the pan and cook for a further 5 minutes. Stir in the parsley just before serving.

Sausage casserole

259 calories

This hearty meal is very filling and is perfect served with some green vegetables, such as curly kale. You can also freeze the casserole in individual portions if you like.

Serves 6   Preparation time: 5 minutes   Cook time: 1¼ hours

1 tsp olive oil (27 cals)

12 low-fat chipolata sausages or 6 sausages (622 cals)

1 onion, peeled and finely chopped (65 cals)

2 garlic cloves, peeled and chopped (6 cals)

1 small carrot, peeled and diced (25 cals)

1 red (bell) pepper, deseeded and diced (51 cals)

1 green (bell) pepper, deseeded and diced (24 cals)

200g (7oz) red lentils (636 cals)

1 chicken stock cube (35 cals)

1 bay leaf

1 × 400g (14oz) can chopped tomatoes (64 cals)

- Heat the olive oil in a medium-sized heavy-based saucepan over a medium heat. Add the sausages and fry until they are tinged with brown, then remove them from the pan and set aside.
- Reduce the heat to low, add the onion, garlic, carrot and (bell) peppers and sauté gently for 5 minutes. Next, stir in the lentils, pour in 1 litre (4 cups) water, then turn the heat to high and bring to the boil. Crumble the stock cube into the pan and add the bay leaf. Reduce the heat to medium and simmer for 10 minutes.
- Reduce the heat, stir in the canned tomatoes, arrange the sausages on the top and cover with a lid. Cook on the lowest heat possible for 40–45 minutes. Alternatively, preheat the oven to 180°C/fan 160°C/350°F/Gas mark 4 and cook in the oven for 1 hour.

Butternut squash with rustic beans and chorizo

281 calories

You can use just cannellini beans instead of the mixed bean salad if you prefer.

Serves 2   Preparation time: 5 minutes   Cook time: 1 hour

1 × 500g (1lb 2oz) butternut squash (180 cals)
2 tsp extra-virgin olive oil (54 cals)
2 garlic cloves, peeled and finely chopped (6 cals)
20g (¾oz) chorizo, diced (58 cals)
2 tbsp tomato purée (paste) (61 cals)
1 × 400g (14oz) can mixed bean salad, rinsed and drained (204 cals)

- Preheat the oven to 210°C/fan 190°C/410°F/Gas mark 6½.
- Cut the squash in half and scoop out and discard the seeds. Using a sharp knife, score the squash flesh deeply at about 1cm (½in) intervals in two directions, making checks or diamonds. The grooves have to reach nearly to the skin or else the squash may not cook through completely. Add 1 teaspoon olive oil to each half and spread over the whole surface with the back of a spoon. Roast in the oven for 1 hour or until cooked.
- Meanwhile, gently heat a small frying pan (skillet), add the garlic and chorizo and fry for 1–2 minutes until both are sizzling and delicious aromas fill the room. Stir in the tomato purée (paste), then add 50ml (scant ¼ cup) water and the beans and stir thoroughly. Bring to a very gentle simmer and cook for 4–5 minutes. If it starts to look dry then just add a little more water.
- Serve the beans piled high on the roasted butternut squash.

Scallops and chipolatas

269 calories

The sausage flavour really complements the scallops.

Serves 1   Preparation time: 1 minute   Cook time: 10 minutes

1 good-quality chipolata sausage (114 cals)

100g (3½oz) small scallops (118 cals)

juice of ½ lime (1 cal)

50g (1¾oz) wild rocket (arugula) (36 cals)

- Cut the chipolata into 1cm (½in) slices. This is easiest with a pair of sharp kitchen scissors.
- Heat a large frying pan (skillet) over a medium heat. When hot, add the chipolata and cook for 6–8 minutes until the sausage slices are cooked through and browning on all sides. The chipolatas will give out some of their fat during cooking so there is no need to add any oil.
- Add the scallops to the pan and fry for 1 minute on each side, then add the lime juice and allow to bubble for a few seconds.
- Place the rocket (arugula) on a serving plate and arrange the scallops and chipolatas over the top, then serve.

Halibut with Parma ham

262 calories

Halibut has a firm, meaty texture that is perfect for this dish. You could also try hake or monkfish.

Serves 2   Preparation time: 5 minutes   Cook time: 10 minutes

2 tsp sunflower oil (54 cals)

2 × 150g (5oz) skinless halibut fillets (276 cals)

2 slices Parma ham (prosciutto) (54 cals)

1 garlic clove, peeled and finely chopped (3 cals)

1 thumb fresh root ginger, peeled and cut into slivers (9 cals)

1 red chilli, deseeded and cut into rings (1 cal)

3 spring onions (scallions), trimmed and shredded (14 cals)

100g (3½oz) mangetout (snow peas), cut in half
on the diagonal (32 cals)

100g (3½oz) broad (fava) beans, podded (59 cals)

1 small pak choi, cut into strips (17 cals)

1 tbsp dark soy sauce (4 cals)

- Heat 1 teaspoon of the oil in a wide frying pan (skillet) until very hot, then add the halibut. Fry for 3–4 minutes on each side until the fish is firm and cooked through.
- Meanwhile, heat the remaining oil in a second frying pan, add the Parma ham (prosciutto) and cook for 1 minute on each side until golden and crisp. Remove from the pan and set aside.
- Add the garlic, ginger and chilli to the pan and fry for 1 minute over a medium heat. Add the spring onions (scallions), mangetout (snow peas) and broad (fava) beans and fry for a further 3–4 minutes, stirring regularly. Finally, add the pak choi and stir-fry for another 2 minutes or until the leaves are wilted.

continued

- Pile the vegetables onto 2 serving plates, place the fish on top and finish with a piece of Parma ham (prosciutto). Drizzle with the soy sauce and serve immediately.

Salmon and cucumber skewers
299 calories

It's best to use metal skewers for this recipe, but if you would like to use wooden ones, be sure to soak them for 30 minutes before using to prevent them burning while cooking.

Serves 1   Preparation time: 5 minutes   Cook time: 10 minutes

1 × 140g (4½oz) skinless, boneless salmon fillet (252 cals)

10cm (4in) piece cucumber, peeled (20 cals)

1 tbsp dark soy sauce (4 cals)

1 tsp runny honey (23 cals)

crisp lettuce leaves, to serve

- Preheat the grill (broiler) to medium-high.
- Using a sharp knife, cut the salmon into 8 roughly equal pieces. Cut the cucumber into 4 rounds, each about 2.5cm (1in) thick, then cut each piece of cucumber in half again to make 8 chunky semi-circles. Alternate the salmon and cucumber pieces onto metal skewers. Start with the salmon, then the cucumber, making sure you go through the outside of the cucumber piece rather than just the fleshy middle.
- Mix the soy sauce and honey together in a small bowl before brushing onto the skewers.
- Place the skewers on the grill pan and grill (broil) for 10 minutes, turning at least once, until the salmon has a crunch to the outside. These skewers also taste delicious barbecued. Serve on a bed of crisp lettuce.

Salmon with lemon mustard sauce

299 calories

The salmon is delicious served with some simple steamed vegetables.

Serves 2   Preparation time: 5 minutes   Cook time: 15 minutes

1 tsp olive oil (27 cals)

2 x 140g (4½oz) skinless salmon fillets (504 cals)

100ml (scant ½ cup) skimmed milk (32 cals)

1 tsp cornflour (cornstarch) (18 cals)

grated zest and juice of ½ lemon (2 cals)

2 tsp Dijon mustard (14 cals)

salt and freshly ground black pepper

1 tsp chopped fresh parsley

- Heat the olive oil in a frying pan over a medium heat. Add the salmon and fry for 4–5 minutes on each side, until just cooked through. Remove from the heat.
- Meanwhile, heat the milk and 50ml (scant ¼ cup) water together in a small saucepan over a high heat. In a small bowl, combine the cornflour (cornstarch) with a little water to make a smooth paste. As the milk starts to boil, slowly drizzle the cornflour paste into the milk, then start whisking the sauce and continue until thickened, about 3–4 minutes. Remove the pan from the heat and stir in the lemon zest and juice, mustard, and a little salt and pepper to taste.
- Place the salmon on 2 serving plates and pour over the sauce. Sprinkle the parsley over the top and serve.

Baked salmon on asparagus

271 calories

Surprisingly simple to put together and quick to cook, this dish is perfect for your fast day.

Serves 1   Preparation time: 5 minutes   Cook time: about 16 minutes, plus 2 minutes resting

1 × 120g (4oz) skinless salmon fillet (216 cals)

1 fresh rosemary sprig

1 fresh sage leaf

4 black peppercorns

1 star anise

½ lemongrass stalk

1 garlic clove, unpeeled and cut in half (3 cals)

2 thick slices lemon

1 tsp olive oil (27 cals)

100g (3½oz) fine asparagus (25 cals)

lemon juice, for drizzling

- Preheat the oven to 190°C/fan 170°C/375°F/Gas mark 5.
- Place a piece of foil on a baking tray and place the salmon in the middle of the foil. Put the rosemary, sage, peppercorns, star anise, lemongrass and garlic around the fish. Put the lemon slices on top and drizzle with the olive oil. Fold the foil around the salmon to make a shallow tent.
- Cook the salmon in the oven for 16 minutes, then remove from the oven and leave to rest for 2 minutes before serving.
- Meanwhile, boil or steam the asparagus for 4–6 minutes, depending on thickness. Arrange the asparagus on a warmed serving plate and place the salmon on top. Drizzle a little lemon juice over the dish and serve.

Tomato and tuna bake

262 calories

This quick and easy one-pot dish is perfect for preparing in advance.

Serves 2   Preparation time: 5 minutes   Cook time: 50 minutes,
plus 10 minutes cooling

180g (6½oz) new potatoes (about 4 medium),
with skin on (126 cals)

1 x 200g (7oz) can tuna steaks in water, drained (148 cals)

1 courgette (zucchini), peeled and finely diced (27 cals)

40 ripe cherry tomatoes, halved (90 cals)

1 garlic clove, peeled and chopped (3 cals)

2 tbsp tomato purée (paste) mixed with 2 tbsp water (61 cals)

1 tsp olive oil (27 cals)

10g (⅓oz) Parmesan cheese, finely grated (42 cals)

salt and freshly ground black pepper

- Boil or steam the new potatoes for 20 minutes until tender, then drain and leave until cool enough to handle.
- Preheat the oven to 190°C/fan 170°C/375°F/Gas mark 5.
- In a small ovenproof baking dish, arrange the tuna, courgette (zucchini) and tomatoes across the bottom, making sure the majority of the tomatoes are cut side up. Sprinkle the chopped garlic over the top, then pour in the tomato purée (paste) mixture.
- When the potatoes are cool, slice them as thinly as possible; the slices should be 2–3mm (¹⁄₁₆–¹⁄₈in) thick. Arrange the potatoes on top of the tuna mixture, allowing them to overlap, then brush the top with the olive oil and sprinkle over the Parmesan and salt and pepper to taste.
- Cook in the oven for 30 minutes, then serve.

Prawn foo young

266 calories

This classic Chinese-Indonesian egg dish can be prepared, cooked and on your plate in less than 15 minutes.

Serves 2   Preparation time: 2 minutes   Cook time: 6 minutes

2 tsp olive oil (54 cals)

3 large free-range eggs, beaten (297 cals)

3 spring onions (scallions), trimmed and shredded (14 cals)

½ garlic clove, peeled and finely chopped (2 cals)

150g (5oz) cooked prawns (shrimp) (148 cals)

1 tbsp dry sherry (14 cals)

1 small handful of fresh coriander (cilantro) leaves, chopped (3 cals)

salt and freshly ground black pepper

- Heat 1 teaspoon of olive oil in a wide saucepan or wok, add the eggs and scramble lightly, removing them from the pan while they are still a little runny and just before they are fully cooked. Transfer to a bowl, cover and set aside.
- Heat the remaining oil, add the spring onions (scallions) and garlic and gently fry for a minute, then add the prawns (shrimp) and fry for a further minute. Add the sherry and coriander (cilantro), season to taste with salt and pepper and stir in the reserved eggs. Cook for a further minute before serving.

Prawn green curry

263 calories

A quick and tasty Thai curry.

Serves 2   Preparation time: 5 minutes   Cook time: 10 minutes

1 tsp sunflower oil (27 cals)

1 tbsp Thai green curry paste (30 cals)

150ml (⅔ cup) vegetable stock, fresh or made
from ¼ stock cube (9 cals)

½ × 400ml (14fl oz) can light coconut milk, stirred (146 cals)

1 red (bell) pepper, deseeded and cut into strips (51 cals)

75g (3oz) frozen peas (50 cals)

1 spring onion (scallion), trimmed and shredded (5 cals)

1 × 160g (5½oz) pak choi, roughly chopped (30 cals)

225g (8oz) raw king prawns (king shrimp) (171 cals)

juice of 1 lime (4 cals)

1 fresh basil leaf, shredded

1 small handful of fresh coriander (cilantro) leaves,
roughly chopped (3 cals)

- Warm the oil in a wide saucepan, add the curry paste and stir-fry for 1 minute before adding the stock and coconut milk. Simmer for 2 minutes, then add the (bell) pepper, peas and spring onion (scallion) and simmer for a further 5 minutes, or until the peas are tender. Add the pak choi and prawns (shrimp) and cook for 2 minutes, or until the prawns turn pink.
- Finally, stir in the lime juice, basil and coriander (cilantro) and serve immediately.

Spicy prawn stir-fry

289 calories

This is a quick and easy meal for one.

Serves 1   Preparation time: 5 minutes   Cook time: about 8 minutes

½ garlic clove, peeled and crushed (2 cals)

½ tsp tamarind paste (6 cals)

1 tbsp dark soy sauce (4 cals)

150g (5oz) cooked king prawns (king shrimp) (148 cals)

½ tsp walnut oil (22 cals)

½ yellow (bell) pepper, deseeded and cut into
thin strips (21 cals)

½ red (bell) pepper, deseeded and cut into
thin strips (51 cals)

1 red chilli, deseeded and cut into fine rings (3 cals)

50g (1¾oz) beansprouts (16 cals)

50g (1¾oz) mangetout (snow peas) (16 cals)

- Mix the garlic, tamarind paste and soy sauce together in a bowl.
  Add the prawns (shrimp) and turn until they are coated all over
  in the dark sticky mixture. Leave to stand for 2 minutes while you
  prepare the rest of the stir-fry.
- Heat the walnut oil in a wok or large frying pan (skillet) over a high
  heat, add the (bell) peppers and chilli and stir-fry for 3 minutes.
  Add the beansprouts and mangetout (snow peas) and stir-fry for
  a further 2 minutes.
- Reduce the heat to medium and add the prawns and marinade
  and stir-fry for a further 2 minutes until the prawns are warmed
  through. Serve immediately.

SNACKS AND SIDES

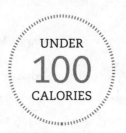

UNDER
100
CALORIES

Virgin Mary

41 calories

Serves 1   Preparation time: 3 minutes

| 4 ice cubes |
| 200ml (generous ¾ cup) tomato juice (28 cals) |
| a pinch of celery salt |
| a pinch of freshly ground black pepper |
| a shake of Tabasco sauce |
| a shake of Worcestershire sauce (1 cal) |
| 1 tsp dry sherry (6 cals) |
| a squeeze of fresh lemon juice (1 cal) |
| 1 short celery stick with leaves, to garnish (5 cals) |

- Put the ice cubes in a long tall glass and pour over the tomato juice. Add the celery salt and pepper, then the Tabasco and Worcestershire sauces. Drizzle in a little dry sherry and a squeeze of lemon juice. Garnish with the celery stick and serve.

Classic salsa

25 calories

This salsa is a million times better than any shop-bought one.

Serves 4   Preparation time: 10 minutes, plus 1 hour standing

¼ red onion, peeled (11 cals)
1 green chilli, deseeded (1 cal)
1 spring onion (scallion) (5 cals)
1 garlic clove, peeled (3 cals)
4 medium tomatoes or 20 cherry tomatoes, cut in half (45 cals)
1 tsp extra-virgin olive oil (27 cals)
a pinch of salt
juice of 1 lemon (4 cals)
1 tsp tomato purée (paste) (5 cals)

- Place the red onion, chilli, spring onion (scallion) and garlic in a food processor and whizz until finely chopped. Add the tomatoes, olive oil, salt, lemon juice, tomato purée (paste) and 1 tablespoon water. Pulse again but leave the tomatoes chunky.
- Transfer to a bowl and check and adjust the salt if necessary. Leave to stand for about 1 hour to allow the flavours to develop. This salsa keeps for up to 3 days in the refrigerator.

White bean hummus

94 calories

This is an interesting variation on traditional hummus. This recipe is most easily made in a food processor. If you prefer, you can make a slightly chunkier hummus by mashing the cannellini beans with a fork instead. This recipe makes six portions and can be kept for up to two days in the refrigerator.

Serves 6   Preparation time: 5 minutes

1 × 400g (14oz) can cannellini beans,
drained and rinsed (259 cals)

2 garlic cloves, peeled (6 cals)

½ tsp ground cumin

¼ tsp paprika (2 cals)

1 tbsp tahini (sesame seed paste) (182 cals)

a pinch of salt

juice of 1 lemon (4 cals)

1 tbsp extra-virgin olive oil (99 cals)

- Place the beans, garlic, cumin, paprika, tahini (sesame seed paste), salt and lemon juice in a food processor and start to whizz. As it starts to clump together, slowly pour the olive oil in through the feed tube. If it's still too thick, add water a little at a time until it reaches the right consistency. Check the seasoning and add more salt if necessary. Transfer the hummus to a large bowl for sharing or place an individual portion (one-sixth) in a small dish.
- Serve with crudités, such as carrot sticks, cucumber, celery and red (bell) pepper, adding on calories appropriately, or with the Homemade Tortilla Chips (see page 192).

Tzatziki

61 calories

Serve with carrot sticks (½ carrot has 18 calories) or strips of red (bell) pepper (1 red pepper has 51 calories).

Serves 1   Preparation time: 5 minutes, plus 1–8 hours chilling

50g (1¾oz) low-fat Greek yogurt (40 cals)
2.5cm (1in) piece cucumber, unpeeled and grated (5 cals)
¼ garlic clove, peeled and crushed (1 cal)
1 tsp fresh lemon juice (1 cal)
½ tsp extra-virgin olive oil (14 cals)
1 tsp chopped fresh dill (optional)
a pinch of salt

- Simply stir all the ingredients together in a bowl, cover and leave to chill in the refrigerator for at least an hour, preferably overnight, before serving.

Coleslaw

83 calories

The easiest method of shredding the cabbage and carrot is to use the grater attachment on a food processor, but it can also be done by hand with a very sharp knife.

Serves 4   Preparation time: 10 minutes

100g (3½oz) low-fat plain yogurt (56 cals)
1 tsp Dijon mustard (7 cals)

3 tbsp extra-light mayonnaise (36 cals)
a pinch of salt
½ white cabbage, shredded (500g/1lb 2oz) (135 cals)
2 carrots, peeled and shredded (70 cals)
½ onion, peeled and very finely chopped (27 cals)

- Mix the yogurt, mustard, mayonnaise and salt together in a large bowl. Add the cabbage, carrots and onion and stir the dressing through thoroughly until the vegetables are coated.
- The coleslaw tastes best if it is left for about an hour before serving. It will also keep for up to 3 days in the refrigerator.

Harissa olives
92 cals

These are a great snack to prepare in advance and keep in a small lidded jar; they are also great for when you're out and about. Try to prepare the olives at least two hours before eating. Serve at room temperature (possibly with a cocktail stick/toothpick!).

Serves 1   Preparation time: 2 minutes, plus 2 hours marinating

16 large black olives (82 cals)
2 tsp good-quality harissa paste (10 cals)

- Place the olives in a small bowl, add the harissa and stir thoroughly. Leave to marinate for at least 2 hours before serving.
- Alternatively, place the olives and harissa in a small lidded jar, shake well and then leave to marinate.

Slow-roasted tomatoes

47 calories

These delicious tomatoes keep for several days in the refrigerator. You can even place a portion in a lidded jar for a quick snack on the go.

Serves 4   Preparation time: 5 minutes   Cook time: 2 hours

500g (1lb 2oz/about 40) ripe and juicy
cherry tomatoes (90 cals)

....

2 tsp sea salt

....

2 fresh rosemary sprigs

....

½ tsp dried mixed herbs

....

1 tbsp extra-virgin olive oil (99 cals)

....

- Preheat the oven to 160°C/fan 140°C/325°F/Gas mark 3.
- Cut the tomatoes in half and place them cut side up in an oven-proof dish. Sprinkle over the salt, rosemary and dried mixed herbs, then drizzle the olive oil over the top.
- Cook the tomatoes in the oven for 2 hours until semi-dried. Leave to cool before serving or packing into a container and chilling in the refrigerator.

Cauliflower pilau rice

34 calories

This tasty 'rice' is made from cauliflower chopped in a food processor and is a great low-calorie alternative to basmati rice. It goes beautifully with any of the curries in this book. You can cook this without the spices if you prefer.

Serves 2   Preparation time: 5 minutes   Cook time: 6–8 minutes

½ small cauliflower (200g/7oz),
cut into small florets (68 cals)

½ tsp cumin seeds

½ tsp coriander seeds

1 cardamom pod

½ tsp turmeric

2 saffron strands

a pinch of salt

- Put the cauliflower florets into a food processor and pulse until the cauliflower is reduced to the size of couscous.
- Crush the cumin seeds, coriander seeds and cardamom pod in a pestle and mortar. Put a medium-sized saucepan with a tight-fitting lid over a high heat and dry-fry the crushed spices for 1 minute. Turn the heat right down and add the cauliflower, 3 tablespoons water and the remaining spices and salt. Stir and cover with the lid. Steam the cauliflower gently for 6 minutes, then check to see if it is tender. It may need 2 minutes more with a little extra water. Serve.

Frozen grapes

36 calories

Because the grapes are frozen they take longer to eat than normal grapes, so they make a great snack.

30 black grapes (36 cals)

- Place the grapes in a small freezerproof container and freeze for at least 2 hours. Remove from the freezer as needed.

Edam and celery

100 calories

A quick-to-put-together snack if you're feeling a little peckish and just can't wait.

Preparation time: 2 minutes

1 × 25g (1oz) slice Edam, cut into 6 strips (85 cals)

3 celery sticks, trimmed and cut in half (15 cals)

sea salt, for dipping

- Place the Edam strips in the centre of each half of the celery. Serve with a little pot of sea salt as a dip.

Melon with Parma ham

78 calories

This is a classic combination.

Serves 1   Preparation time: 2 minutes

¼ Galia melon (100g/3½oz), deseeded (24 cals)
2 slices Parma ham (prosciutto) (54 cals)

- Cut the melon in half again so you have 2 slices, still in the skin. Using a sharp knife, cut the melon just inside the skin but leave it in place, then cut into small chunks.
- Cut the Parma ham (prosciutto) into small pieces using kitchen scissors. Sprinkle the ham over the melon and serve.

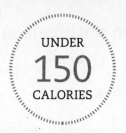

UNDER
150
CALORIES

Cottage cheese with peaches

115 calories

This tasty quick snack is perfect for your fast day.

Preparation time: 2 minutes

100g (3½oz) low-fat cottage cheese (79 cals)

1 medium ripe peach, pitted and cut into eighths (36 cals)

- Pile the cottage cheese on a small plate and arrange the peach over the top and eat.

Homemade tortilla chips

118 calories

Crisps (potato chips) are my secret indulgence, and I really shouldn't eat them! These tortilla chips are delicious, especially served with the Classic salsa (see page 184), and help satisfy my need for crisps.

Serves 1   Preparation time: 2 minutes   Cook time: 5 minutes

1 tortilla wrap (118 cals – but check the packet,
the calories can vary)

salt and freshly ground black pepper

- Preheat the oven to 220°C/fan 200°C/425°F/Gas mark 7.
- Cut the tortilla wrap into small triangles, place on a non-stick baking tray and sprinkle on a little salt and pepper. Cook in the oven for 4–5 minutes until just starting to brown.
- Leave to cool completely on the baking tray before transferring to a bowl before serving.

Garlic and Parmesan popcorn
130 calories

This is another quick and easy snack. Be sure to move the pan while the corn is popping to prevent it from burning.

Serves 1   Preparation time: 1 minute   Cook time: 4 minutes

½ tsp sunflower oil (14 cals)

½ garlic clove, peeled and crushed (2 cals)

20g (¾oz) uncooked popping corn (72 cals)

10g (⅓oz) Parmesan cheese, finely grated (42 cals)

a pinch of salt

a pinch of cayenne pepper

- Heat the oil and garlic in a small lidded saucepan. When the oil is hot, add the popping corn, cover with the lid and cook over a high heat for 1 minute. When the corn begins to pop, move the pan back and forth over the heat until the popping subsides. Remove the pan from the heat and carefully remove the lid – some corn may still pop. Add the Parmesan, salt and cayenne, toss to coat, then transfer to a bowl to serve.

TREATS AND PUDDINGS

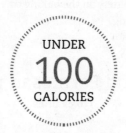

UNDER
100
CALORIES

Mint tea

4 calories

As this is practically calorie free, I often have a pot or two on a fasting day, made with fresh mint from the garden. It can also be served with a teaspoon of honey if preferred, which adds 25 calories.

Serves 1   Preparation time: 2 minutes, plus 5–7 minutes infusing

1 handful of fresh mint leaves,
roughly chopped (4 cals)

- Fill a small teapot with boiling water and add the mint leaves. Leave to steep for 5–7 minutes. Strain the tea into a cup or heat-proof glass and drink.

Tropical juice smoothie
86 calories

This is a refreshing pick-me-up juice.

Serves 1   Preparation time: 2 minutes

5 tbsp unsweetened pineapple juice (31 cals)

5 tbsp unsweetened orange juice (27 cals)

5 tbsp unsweetened apple juice (28 cals)

4–5 ice cubes

- Pour all the juices into a blender, add the ice cubes and blend. Pour into a glass and drink.

Summer fruit sorbet
93 calories

A refreshing dessert with such a low calorie count that you can keep it in the freezer and treat yourself on a fasting day.

*Serves 6   Preparation time: 10 minutes, plus 2 hours standing
and 1–4 hours freezing*

500g (1lb 2oz) frozen summer fruit mix (raspberries, blackberries, blackcurrants, etc.) (240 cals)

4 tbsp granulated sugar (315 cals)

juice of 1 lemon (4 cals)

- Place the still-frozen berries in a wide bowl and sprinkle with the sugar and lemon juice. Cover and leave to defrost fully for at least 2 hours.   *continued*

- Uncover the fruits and mash gently with a fork. Place in a sieve (strainer) over a large bowl and squeeze all the juice through, discarding the remaining pulp.
- Transfer to an ice-cream machine and churn for about 1 hour or until the desired consistency is achieved, then place in a freezerproof container and freeze until needed. Alternatively, if you don't have an ice-cream machine, transfer the liquid straight to a freezerproof container and freeze. After 30 minutes take the sorbet out of the freezer and mash it with a fork to remove any ice crystals, then return it to the freezer. Repeat this process every 30 minutes until frozen. It will take about 4 hours to freeze completely.

Peach sorbet
63 calories

Keep this sorbet in the freezer especially for fasting days.

Serves 6 Preparation time: 5 minutes, plus 1–4 hours freezing

2 level tbsp granulated sugar (158 cals)
....
6 ripe peaches, peeled and stoned (pitted) (218 cals)
....

- Place the sugar in a cup, pour on a little boiling water and stir until dissolved.
- Place the peach flesh in a food processor and whizz until smooth, then transfer to a bowl and add the sugar syrup. Mix, then pour the peaches through a sieve (strainer) into another bowl. Press gently against the sieve with a fork to make as much of the juice go through as possible. Discard the flesh and transfer the juice to an ice-cream machine. Churn until the correct consistency is achieved, then place in a freezerproof container and freeze.
- If you don't have an ice-cream machine, transfer the juice to a freezerproof container and put into the freezer. After 30 minutes take the sorbet out of the freezer and mash it with a fork to remove any ice crystals, then return it to the freezer. Repeat this process every 30 minutes until frozen. It will take about 4 hours to freeze completely.

Watermelon sherbet

80 calories

This light and airy mix of frozen watermelon and yogurt makes a refreshing dessert. It is most easily made with an ice-cream machine, but I have also included instructions for making it without one.

Serves 6 Preparation time: 20 minutes, plus 1–4 hours freezing
Cook time: about 5 minutes, plus 20 minutes cooling

50g (1¾oz) caster (superfine) sugar (197 cals)

1 normal-sized watermelon, flesh only (600g/1¼lb),
deseeded and diced (186 cals)

100g (3½oz) low-fat Greek yogurt (80 cals)

1 tsp vanilla extract (12 cals)

juice of 1 lime (4 cals)

- Heat the sugar and 50ml (scant ¼ cup) water in a small saucepan over a medium heat and cook, stirring constantly, until the sugar is dissolved. Remove from the heat and leave to cool.
- Put the watermelon into a blender and pulse until smooth. Depending on the size of the blender, you'll need to do this in several batches. Transfer the watermelon to a large bowl and stir in the sugar syrup, yogurt, vanilla extract and lime juice. Pour the mixture through a sieve (strainer) into another bowl, pressing the watermelon gently to release all the juice, and discard the pulp.
- Transfer the mixture to an ice-cream machine and churn for about 1 hour or until frozen and a 'soft serve' consistency. Place the sherbet in a freezerproof container and freeze until needed. Alternatively, transfer the mixture to a freezerproof container and freeze. After 30 minutes take the sherbet out of the freezer and mash it with a fork to remove any ice crystals, then return it to the freezer. Repeat this process every 30 minutes until frozen. It will take about 4 hours to freeze completely. Remove from the freezer about 10 minutes before serving.

Pears poached in lemonade

66 calories

Serves 1   Preparation time: 2 minutes   Cook time: 8 minutes

1 hard dessert pear, peeled, cored and
cut into quarters (60 cals)

200ml (generous ¾ cup) diet lemonade (6 cals)

- Place the pear quarters in a small saucepan and cover with the lemonade. Bring to a simmer and cook for 8 minutes. Alternatively, place the pears and lemonade in a microwaveable bowl and cook in the microwave for 8 minutes.

Strawberries with toasted almonds and ginger

89 calories

When the strawberries are prepared in this way they make a brilliant strawberry syrup.

Serves 4   Preparation time: 10 minutes, plus 10 minutes standing

250g (9oz) strawberries, hulled (68 cals)

10 whole almonds (122 cals)

50ml (scant ¼ cup) fresh unsweetened orange juice (18 cals)

1 tbsp crystallized ginger, chopped (69 cals)

1 level tbsp caster (superfine) sugar (79 cals)

- Cut the strawberries into slices, about 5mm (¼in) thick, then use a sharp knife to roughly chop the almonds. Put the almonds in a small frying pan (skillet) and dry-fry over a medium heat for 2–4 minutes, stirring frequently, until fragrant and lightly browned. Remove from the heat and set aside.

- Combine the strawberries, orange juice, ginger and caster (superfine) sugar in a large bowl. Stir and leave to stand at room temperature for 10 minutes.
- When you are ready to serve, divide the strawberries into 4 small bowls and sprinkle with the toasted almonds.

Perfect meringues

57 calories per meringue

There is a bit of an art to this recipe, but it is well worth the effort.

Makes 20 meringues   Preparation time: 15 minutes   Cook time: 6 hours

1 lemon, cut in half
....
5 egg whites, at room temperature (45 cals)
....
300g (11oz) golden caster (superfine) sugar (1086 cals)
....

- Preheat the oven to 200°C/fan 180°C/400°F/Gas mark 6 and line a baking sheet (cookie sheet) with greaseproof (waxed) paper.
- Wipe a large bowl and the whisk with the cut side of the lemon. They need to be meticulously clean for the egg whites to whisk up well and the lemon juice helps this. Add the egg whites to the bowl and, using an electric mixer, whisk until stiff peaks form. While whisking, spoon in the sugar a tablespoon at a time. Firm peaks should be maintained. Finally, add a squeeze of lemon juice to help them keep their shape.
- Spoon small blobs of the whisked egg whites onto the prepared baking sheet, then place in the oven and switch the oven off immediately. Do not open the oven door. Leave the meringues to cook in the slowly cooling oven for about 6 hours or overnight.

Chocolate meringue biscuits

21 calories per biscuit

Once cool, store these biscuits (cookies) in an airtight container. They will keep for 3–4 days.

Makes 24 biscuits   Preparation time: 10 minutes
Cook time: 1½ hours, plus 2 hours cooling

3 tbsp cocoa powder (unsweetened cocoa) (140 cals),
plus 1 tsp for dusting (6 cals)

75g (3oz) caster (superfine) sugar (296 cals)

6 egg whites at room temperature (54 cals)

a small pinch of salt

¼ tsp cream of tartar (2 cals)

1 tsp vanilla extract (12 cals)

⅛ tsp ground cinnamon, for dusting

- Preheat the oven to 130°C/fan 110°C/250°F/Gas mark ½ and line two baking sheets (cookie sheets) with greaseproof (waxed) paper.
- In a small bowl, mix the cocoa and caster (superfine) sugar together.
- Put the egg whites into a large, clean, dry bowl and, using an electric mixer, whisk the egg whites until foamy. While whisking, add the salt, cream of tartar and vanilla extract, then add the cocoa and sugar mixture 1 tablespoon at a time. Whisk the mixture until it forms stiff peaks.
- Drop tablespoonfuls of the mixture onto the prepared baking sheets.
- Put the 1 teaspoon cocoa and the cinnamon into a small sieve (strainer) and dust the biscuits with the mixture. Bake in the oven for 1½ hours, then turn off the oven and leave the biscuits (cookies) to cool in the oven with the door slightly ajar for another 2 hours.
- When the biscuits are cold, remove them from the oven and store in an airtight container.

Date and coconut cookies

81 calories per cookie

These moreish cookies are very easy to make.

Makes 24 cookies   Preparation time: 10 minutes   Cook time: 10 minutes, plus 30 minutes chilling

25g (1oz) butter (186 cals)

100g (3½oz) caster (superfine) sugar (394 cals)

250g (9oz) pitted dates, finely chopped (675 cals)

½ tsp vanilla extract (6 cals)

100g (3½oz) Rice Krispies (382 cals)

50g (1¾oz) desiccated (dry unsweetened) coconut (302 cals)

- Combine the butter, sugar and dates in a large saucepan and cook over a gentle heat until the butter is melted and the dates are mostly dissolved, about 10 minutes.
- Take the pan off the heat and add the vanilla extract, Rice Krispies and coconut. Stir well, then leave in the pan until just cool enough to handle.
- Line a baking sheet (cookie tray) with greaseproof (waxed) paper. Roll teaspoons of the mixture to make 2.5cm (1in) diameter balls and place them on the prepared baking sheet, flattening them slightly with the palm of your hand. Chill in the refrigerator for about 30 minutes, or until firm.

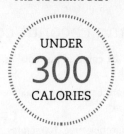

UNDER

300

CALORIES

Raspberry frozen yogurt

146 calories

A great fat-free dessert, it is made without the use of an ice-cream machine. Remember to take the frozen yogurt out of the freezer 10 minutes before serving to allow it to soften slightly. Feel free to experiment with other fruits using a similar method, or try adding a few drops of vanilla extract to make vanilla frozen yogurt.

Serves 6   Preparation time: 10 minutes, plus 3–4 hours freezing

200g (7oz) raspberries (50 cals)

½ × 400ml (14fl oz) can light condensed milk (541 cals)

500g (1lb 2oz) pot zero fat Greek yogurt (285 cals)

- Roughly chop half the raspberries and set aside.
- Place the remaining raspberries in a food processor and whizz to a smooth purée. Alternatively, purée the raspberries with a fork.
- Place the puréed raspberries in a large bowl and stir in the condensed milk and Greek yogurt until everything is mixed, then fold in the remaining chopped raspberries. Transfer the mixture to a freezerproof container and freeze until solid.

Raspberry cream

108 calories

This dessert is also delicious prepared with fresh cherries (48 calories for 100g/3½oz).

Serves 2   Preparation time: 5 minutes   Cook time: 7 minutes, plus 20 minutes cooling

1 level tbsp caster (superfine) sugar (79 cals)

150g (5oz) fresh raspberries (38 cals)

50g (1¾oz) light sweetened aerosol cream (98 cals)

- Place 4 tablespoons water and the sugar in a small saucepan and bring to the boil. Boil for 2 minutes, then reduce the heat and stir in the raspberries, setting aside a small handful for decoration. Cook gently for 5 minutes, then remove the pan from the heat and leave to cool.
- Transfer the raspberry mixture to a blender and whizz until smooth, or mash with a fork. Fold in the cream, then divide the mixture between 2 small bowls and serve with the reserved raspberries scattered over the top.

Boozy plums and apples
136 calories

This quick and easy dessert can be served hot or cold.

Serves 6   Preparation time: 10 minutes   Cook time: 5 minutes

8 plums, stoned (pitted) and chopped (158 cals)

4 large eating apples, peeled, cored and
thinly sliced (288 cals)

200ml (generous ¾ cup) good-quality
dry (hard) cider (72 cals)

75g (3oz) caster (superfine) sugar (296 cals)

¼ tsp ground cinnamon

- Combine all the ingredients in a saucepan. Bring to a simmer over a medium heat, cover with a lid and cook, stirring every minute, for 5 minutes until the fruit is tender.

Classic baked apple
186 calories

Be sure to score a line round the middle of the apple before filling, otherwise it may split during cooking.

Serves 1   Preparation time: 5 minutes   Cook time: 35–40 minutes

1 large Bramley (cooking) apple (54 cal)

1 tsp butter (37 cals)

1 tsp flaked (slivered) almonds (32 cals)

2 tsp soft dark brown sugar (36 cals)

½ tsp ground mixed spice

10g (¼oz) raisins (27 cals)

grated zest of ½ orange

- Preheat the oven to 190°C/fan 170°C/375°F/Gas mark 5.
- Use an apple corer to remove the core from the apple, then score round the middle of the apple with a sharp knife, cutting to a depth of about 5mm (¼in) all round. Place the apple in a small overproof serving dish.
- Mix the rest of the ingredients together in a small bowl and use to stuff the filling into the centre, rubbing a little round the apple as well. If there is any filling left over, pile it on the top. Cook in the oven for 35–40 minutes until golden and soft.

Stewed rhubarb

158 calories

This is a simple fat-free pudding, perfect for your fast day.

Serves 4   Preparation time: 5 minutes   Cook time: 12 minutes

500g (1lb 2oz) rhubarb, trimmed and cut into
3cm (1¼in) slices (35 cals)

150g (5oz) caster (superfine) sugar (591 cals)

juice of 1 lemon (4 cals)

- Place the rhubarb, sugar, 2 tablespoons water and the lemon juice in a medium-sized saucepan. Cover with a lid and cook over a low heat for 12 minutes, stirring occasionally, until tender. Serve.

Chocolate strawberry lollies

116 calories

These lollies are just a little bit of fun and look very retro.

Serves 1   Preparation time: 10 minutes, plus 30 minutes chilling

about 10 medium strawberries, hulled (40 cals)

½ orange (decorative!)

15g (½oz) plain (semisweet) chocolate, broken
into pieces (76 cals)

- Cut any large strawberries in half, then wash and dry on kitchen paper (paper towels). Place the orange half upside down on a small plate.
- Melt the chocolate in a small heatproof bowl set over a saucepan of gently simmering water. It will melt in about a minute. Remove the pan from the heat.
- Put a cocktail stick (toothpick) in the fat end of each strawberry and dip the tip into the melted chocolate, then place the cocktail stick in the orange so the strawberry is pointing out. Repeat with the other strawberries, arranging them decoratively round the orange as you go. Leave in the refrigerator for about 30 minutes until set.

Cocoa and raisin cereal bars

143 calories

These bars are very filling and can last for at least a week in an airtight container.

Serves 16   Preparation time: 10 minutes, plus 15 minutes soaking
Cook time: 45 minutes, plus 15 minutes cooling

100g (3½oz) raisins (272 cals)

low-cal spray oil, for oiling

1 x 400ml (14fl oz) can light condensed milk (1068 cals)

20g (¾oz) cocoa powder
(unsweetened cocoa) (62 cals)

250g (9oz) porridge (rolled) oats (890 cals)

a few drops of vanilla extract

- Place the raisins in a small bowl and pour on boiling water so that it just covers the raisins. Leave to soak for about 15 minutes.
- Preheat the oven to 160°C/fan 140°C/325°F/Gas mark 3 and line the base of a 20cm (8in) square cake tin (pan) with greaseproof (waxed) paper. Spray with low-cal oil spray to prevent the oats sticking to the paper.
- Warm the condensed milk in a small saucepan over a low heat for about 5 minutes. Don't boil.
- Put the cocoa in a cup, add a little just-boiled water and stir to make a thin paste.
- Place the oats in a large bowl. Remove the condensed milk from the heat and stir in the cocoa paste, raisins and vanilla extract. Pour the mixture over the oats, mix thoroughly, then spoon into the prepared cake tin and bake in the oven for 45 minutes.
- When cooked, immediately remove from the tin and transfer to a chopping (cutting) board. Cut into 16 squares with a very sharp knife, then leave to cool completely on the board before transferring to an airtight tin.

Beetroot and chocolate cupcakes

120 calories per cake

These squidgy cupcakes make a delicious treat. If you've never tried the beetroot and chocolate combination before, you will be blown away by how good they are.

Makes 24 cupcakes   Preparation time: 20 minutes
Cook time: 20 minutes, plus 15 minutes cooling

3 large free-range eggs (272 cals)
150g (5oz) caster (superfine) sugar (591 cals)
200g (7oz) raw beetroot, peeled and finely grated (72 cals)
280ml (1¼ cups) buttermilk (104 cals)
½ tsp vanilla extract (6 cals)
180g (6¼oz) plain (all-purpose) flour, sifted (614 cals)
180g (6¼oz) ground almonds (1102 cals)
2 level tsp baking powder (14 cals)
2 tbsp cocoa powder (unsweetened cocoa) (94 cals)

- Preheat the oven to 190°C/fan 170°C/375°F/Gas mark 5 and line two bun tins (muffin pans) with paper cases.
- In a large mixing bowl, whisk together the eggs and sugar until light and fluffy. This is easiest with an electric mixer but a hand whisk is fine. Stir in the beetroot, buttermilk and vanilla extract, then fold in the flour, ground almonds, baking powder and cocoa.
- Divide the batter between the paper cases and bake in the oven for 20 minutes or until the cakes spring back lightly when pressed with a finger. Remove the cupcakes from the tin and leave to cool on a wire rack.

Vanilla custard dessert

170 calories

This vanilla custard can be eaten immediately or chilled in the refrigerator to make a cold dessert, if you like.

Serves 4   Preparation time: 10 minutes   Cook time 10 minutes

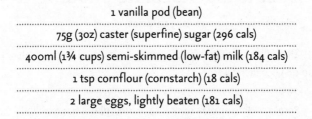

1 vanilla pod (bean)
....
75g (3oz) caster (superfine) sugar (296 cals)
....
400ml (1¾ cups) semi-skimmed (low-fat) milk (184 cals)
....
1 tsp cornflour (cornstarch) (18 cals)
....
2 large eggs, lightly beaten (181 cals)
....

- Split the vanilla pod (bean) in half lengthways and scrape out the seeds with a knife. Set aside 4 teaspoons of the sugar.
- Put 250ml (generous 1 cup) of the milk in a large saucepan over a medium heat with the vanilla pod (bean) and seeds. Heat until steaming. Do not boil. Remove the vanilla pod from the saucepan.
- Mix the remaining sugar and cornflour (cornstarch) together in a large bowl. Add the eggs and whisk until smooth, then slowly add the remaining milk, whisking all the time until fully combined and smooth.
- Pour the egg mixture slowly into the saucepan and continue to whisk constantly over a medium heat until thickened, about 3 minutes.
- Divide the mixture between 4 ramekins or small glasses, then sprinkle a teaspoon of the reserved sugar over each dish. Serve.

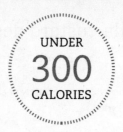

UNDER
300
CALORIES

Low-fat chocolate pudding

255 calories

This healthy dessert is ideal for when you are in need of a chocolate pick-me-up on your fast day.

Serves 4   Preparation time: 10 minutes, plus 4 hours chilling

450ml (2 cups) whole milk (297 cals)

15g/½oz butter (112 cals)

100g (3½oz) caster (superfine) sugar (394 cals)

2 level tbsp cocoa powder (unsweetened cocoa) (62 cals)

2 level tbsp cornflour (cornstarch) (142 cals)

1 tsp vanilla extract (12 cals)

- Heat the milk and butter together in a medium-sized saucepan over a gentle heat until the butter has melted. Set aside 4 teaspoons of the sugar and stir the rest into the pan until dissolved.
- Meanwhile, place the cocoa, cornflour (cornstarch) and 2 tablespoons water in a small bowl and stir well to make a smooth paste.
- Pour the paste gradually into the saucepan, whisking constantly. Continue to whisk while you increase the heat to high and cook until thick and bubbly, about 5 minutes. Remove the pan from the heat and stir in the vanilla extract.
- Spoon the mixture into 4 ramekins or small glasses and sprinkle a teaspoon of the reserved sugar over each one (this prevents a skin from forming). Leave to cool, then cover with cling film (plastic wrap) and chill in the refrigerator for about 4 hours until set.

PART 4

EXERCISE

INTRODUCTION

In buying this book and following the 5:2 Bikini Diet you have taken the first step to improving your body and health. If you really want to achieve amazing results fast, then take the next step and combine your diet with a targeted and accessible exercise programme. The following 30-day training plan has been designed by David Jones, founder of Sculpt Health and Fitness: **www.sculpt.me.uk**.

The Sculpt team has helped countless people get into the best shape through expert coaching and focused health and fitness programmes. No matter how much weight you think you have got to lose, and even if you haven't exercised for 20 years – or ever at all – this programme can help you. We have helped mums feel confident enough in their bodies to wear a bikini for the first time since their twenties; we have helped men turn their beer guts into six packs. Anyone can follow this exercise plan; no matter what barriers you think might be in your way, you can be active and accelerate the results you will see through following the 5:2 Bikini Diet.

The 12 simple-to-follow workouts on pages 217–23 go hand in hand with the 5:2 Bikini Diet and are designed to burn as much body fat as possible while improving muscle tone, strength, fitness and posture. They don't involve endless hours of jogging and you don't have to be a member of a gym. The beauty of the Sculpt 30 plan is that it can be done in whatever environment you feel most comfortable, whether that's your own home, a park or in a gym. The plan uses an incredibly effective combination of resistance training (for your muscles) and cardio intervals to raise your body's in-built fat-burning device – your metabolism. Each one of these 12 workouts will raise your metabolism for up to 24 hours after finishing the session, leaving you with a leaner, healthier body in just 30 days.

To ensure the best results, follow these golden rules:

Be consistent

When it comes to exercise and diet, you get out what you put in. If you fully commit to the 5:2 Bikini Diet and the Sculpt 30 programme, you can expect great results in just 30 days. If you follow the plan 70 per cent of the time, you can expect okay results. If you cheat on your diet and skip training sessions regularly, you are severely damaging your chances of getting your beach-ready body.

Make it part of your routine

We are habitual creatures, so make your three weekly sessions part of your regular schedule, write them into your diary and don't let anything interfere with them.

Set a goal

It could be to lose a few pounds, it may be to look great in your bikini on holiday. Pick something that motivates you and focus all of your diet and training efforts on achieving it.

Apply yourself

If you go through the motions when training or don't progress your efforts as you get fitter and stronger, your results will plateau. Aim to improve something every session: it could be the amount of weight lifted, the difficulty of the exercise or reduced rest periods.

Measure your success

If you are not assessing, you are guessing. On the same day and at the same time once a week, weigh yourself, take waist, thigh, hip, chest and arm measurements, take a photo of yourself and ideally get your body fat percentage taken by a professional (the body fat calculators on scales are often inaccurate).

Get some support

Find a friend with similar goals to follow the programme with you. Tell your partner, family, friends and colleagues what you are trying to achieve and ask for their support.

Train your mind as well as your body

A positive frame of mind is essential for great results; as soon as you let negativity creep in it will be all too easy to fall off the wagon or even give up completely. Keep the focus on your goal and how much you want to achieve it.

HOW TO GET STARTED

Sculpt strongly recommends that you consult with your doctor before beginning any exercise programme. You should understand that when participating in any exercise or programme, there is the possibility of physical injury. If you engage in this exercise programme, you agree that you do so at your own risk.

The Sculpt 30 programme comprises of 12 training sessions over a four-week period that get progressively more difficult. For best results you should complete three sessions per week. Sessions should not be done on consecutive days or on your fasting days, as you may be low on energy.

The plan has been designed using minimal equipment so it can be undertaken at home or in a park, but of course it can also be completed in a gym. If training at home, you will need:

- an exercise mat
- an adjustable dumbbell set with weights
- resistance bands
- a Swiss ball
- an adjustable step or bench

Before starting a session it's very important to warm up correctly. This will prepare your body for the task at hand and will help to avoid any injuries. Likewise, after every session it's important to stretch the muscles you have been working to avoid them tightening between sessions. See pages 216–7 for detailed instructions on how to warm up and stretch correctly.

To maximize results and fat-burning potential, the Sculpt 30 plan uses a combination of resistance exercises (exercises for your muscles), completed in superset fashion (two or more sets completed consecutively with minimal rest in between). The supersets are labelled A1, A2 and A3, and to perform them correctly just complete the given sets and repetitions (reps) for exercise A1, then immediately move on to A2 and A3 until all sets are completed. Then take a short rest before moving on to supersets B1, B2 and B3.

Every Sculpt 30 session is finished with a short blast of cardio interval training (labelled C1), as cardio intervals have been proven to raise metabolism and greatly increase fat-burning potential.

When performing all reps and sets of any given exercise, make sure to concentrate on holding the perfect technique and think about the muscles that you are using. In doing this you will increase the effectiveness of your sessions and accelerate results. It's also important to perform exercises at the correct tempo, as rushing reduces effectiveness. For every exercise follow a 3-1-1 tempo, i.e. simply lower the weight for 3 seconds, hold the bottom position for 1 second and then lift the weight in 1 second.

If you are unsure how to execute any of the exercises, refer to the guide on pages 224–32. You can also find visual demonstrations of all the exercises in this plan on the Sculpt YouTube channel at **www.sculpt.me.uk**. For more advanced participants, the guide has progressions included for all exercises given in the plan.

How to warm up and cool down

Warming up correctly is absolutely essential before starting all 12 of the Sculpt 30 workouts. Warming up prepares your body and mind for a tough and effective session and without it you will reduce your chances of getting great results. You will also run the risk of sustaining an injury, thereby completely derailing your exercise efforts. Before every session, complete the following simple warm-up routine (an explanation of each exercise is contain on pages 224–32):

- Squat with arms stretched above your head x 10 reps
- Hold your arms out to your sides and rotate your body x 10 reps
- On the spot alternately march a knee high to your chest x 20 reps
- On a mat, perform a plank for 30 seconds, engaging your abs
- Lying on your back, perform 15 hip bridges, squeezing your bottom
- Knee press-ups x 10 reps
- Star jumps x 30 reps
- On the spot, swing each leg x 10 reps
- Walking lunges x 10 reps
- Rotate your arms forwards and backwards x 10 reps

After completing each session, it's also important to stretch the muscles you have been using to avoid them getting too tight:

- Hamstring stretch × 20 seconds each leg
- Quad stretch × 20 seconds each leg
- Calf muscle stretch × 20 seconds
- Chest and shoulder stretch × 20 seconds
- Lower-back stretch × 20 seconds

If you are unsure how to perform any of the exercises or stretches, refer to the guide on pages 224–32 or check out the Sculpt YouTube channel at **www.sculpt.me.uk**

Week 1: Session 1

(Warm up) A detailed explanation of all the exercises is given in the exercise guide on pages 224–32.

Superset	Exercise	Sets	Reps	Tempo	Rest
A1	Body weight squats	3	10	3-1-1	0
A2	Knee press-ups	3	10	3-1-1	0
A3	Plank	3	30 secs	-	60 secs
B1	High step-ups	3	10 each leg	3-1-1	0
B2	Upright rows	3	10	3-1-1	0
B3	Hip bridges	3	15	3-1-1	60 secs
C1	Fast step-ups	8	30 secs	Fast!	60 secs

(Stretch)

Week 1: Session 2

(Warm up)

Superset	Exercise	Sets	Reps	Tempo	Rest
A1	Dumbbell deadlifts	3	10	3-1-1	0
A2	Dumbbell chest press	3	10	3-1-1	0
A3	Mountain climbers	3	20	1-1-1	60 secs
B1	Walking lunges	3	10 each leg	3-1-1	0
B2	Dumbbell lat pull overs	3	10	3-1-1	0
B3	Cobras	3	15	3-1-1	60 secs
C1	Fast run	8	30 secs	Fast!	60 secs

(Stretch)

Week 1: Session 3

(Warm up)

Superset	Exercise	Sets	Reps	Tempo	Rest
A1	Dumbbell squat-curl press	3	12	3-1-1	0
A2	Knee press-ups	3	10	3-1-1	0
A3	Heel taps	3	20	1-1-1	60 secs
B1	Reverse lunge knee lifts	3	10 each leg	3-1-1	0
B2	Dumbbell single arm rows	3	10 each arm	3-1-1	0
B3	Ab crunches	3	15	3-1-1	60 secs
C1	Burpees	8	30 secs	Fast!	60 secs

(Stretch)

Week 2: Session 4

(Warm up)

Superset	Exercise	Sets	Reps	Tempo	Rest
A1	Dumbbell squats	3	12	3-1-1	0
A2	Knee press-ups	3	12	3-1-1	0
A3	Side planks	3	40 secs	-	60 secs
B1	Dumbbell high step-ups	3	12 each leg	3-1-1	0
B2	Upright rows	3	12	3-1-1	0
B3	Single leg hip bridges	3	15 each leg	3-1-1	60 secs
C1	Fast step-ups	10	30 secs	Fast!	60 secs

(Stretch)

Week 2: Session 5

(Warm up)

Superset	Exercise	Sets	Reps	Tempo	Rest
A1	Dumbbell deadlifts	3	12	3-1-1	0
A2	Dumbbell chest press	3	12	3-1-1	0
A3	Squat thrusts	3	24	1-1-1	60 secs
B1	Walking dumbbell lunges	3	12 each leg	3-1-1	0
B2	Dumbbell lat pull overs	3	12	3-1-1	0
B3	Cobras	3	15	3-1-1	60 secs
C1	Fast run	10	30 secs	Fast!	90 secs

(Stretch)

Week 2: Session 6

(Warm up)

Superset	Exercise	Sets	Reps	Tempo	Rest
A1	Dumbbell squat-curl press	3	12	3-1-1	0
A2	Knee press-ups	3	12	3-1-1	0
A3	Heel taps	3	24	1-1-1	60 secs
B1	Dumbbell reverse lunge knee lifts	3	12 each leg	3-1-1	0
B2	Bent over dumbbell rows	3	12 each arm	3-1-1	0
B3	Ab crunches	3	15	3-1-1	60 secs
C1	Burpees	10	30 secs	Fast!	90 secs

(Stretch)

Week 2: Session 7

(Warm up)

Superset	Exercise	Sets	Reps	Tempo	Rest
A1	Dumbbell squat & shoulder press	3	15	3-1-1	0
A2	Press-ups	3	15	3-1-1	0
A3	Side planks	3	40 secs	-	60 secs
B1	Dumbbell high step-up & bicep curl	3	15 each leg	3-1-1	0
B2	Upright rows	3	15	3-1-1	0
B3	Swiss ball hip bridges	3	15	3-1-1	60 secs
C1	Fast step-ups	8	40 secs	Fast!	60 secs

(Stretch)

Week 3: Session 8

(Warm up)

Superset	Exercise	Sets	Reps	Tempo	Rest
A1	Dumbbell deadlifts	3	15	3-1-1	0
A2	Swiss ball dumbbell chest press	3	15	3-1-1	0
A3	Swiss ball mountain climbers	3	20	1-1-1	60 secs
B1	Walking body weight lunges & bicep curl	3	15 each leg	3-1-1	0
B2	Dumbbell lat pull overs	3	15	3-1-1	0
B3	Swiss ball cobras	3	15	3-1-1	60 secs
C1	Fast run	8	40 secs	Fast!	90 secs

(Stretch)

Week 3: Session 9

(Warm up)

Superset	Exercise	Sets	Reps	Tempo	Rest
A1	Dumbbell squat-curl press	3	15	3-1-1	0
A2	Press-ups	3	15	3-1-1	0
A3	Heel taps	3	30	1-1-1	60 secs
B1	Dumbbell reverse lunge knee lifts	3	15 each leg	3-1-1	0
B2	Dumbbell single arm rows	3	15 each arm	3-1-1	0
B3	Swiss ball ab crunches	3	15	3-1-1	60 secs
C1	Burpees	8	40 secs	Fast!	90 secs

(Stretch)

Week 4: Session 10

(Warm up)

Superset	Exercise	Sets	Reps	Tempo	Rest
A1	Dumbbell squats	4	10	3-1-1	0
A2	Press-ups	4	10	3-1-1	0
A3	Swiss ball plank	4	30 secs	-	60 secs
B1	Dumbbell high step-ups	4	10 each leg	3-1-1	0
B2	Upright rows	4	10	3-1-1	0
B3	Swiss ball hip bridges	4	15	3-1-1	60 secs
C1	Fast step-ups	10	30 secs	Fast!	60 secs

(Stretch)

Week 4: Session 11

(Warm up)

Superset	Exercise	Sets	Reps	Tempo	Rest
A1	Dumbbell deadlifts	4	10	3-1-1	0
A2	Swiss ball dumbbell press	4	10	3-1-1	0 chest
A3	Squat thrusts	4	20	1-1-1	60 secs
B1	Walking dumbbell lunges	4	10 each leg	3-1-1	0
B2	Dumbbell lat pull overs	4	10	3-1-1	0
B3	Swiss ball cobras	3	15	3-1-1	60 secs
C1	Fast run	10	30 secs	Fast!	90 secs

(Stretch)

Week 4: Session 12

(Warm up)

Superset	Exercise	Sets	Reps	Tempo	Rest
A1	Dumbbell squat-curl press	4	10	3-1-1	0
A2	Press-ups	4	10	3-1-1	0
A3	Heel taps	4	20	1-1-1	60 secs
B1	Dumbbell reverse lunge knee lifts	4	10 each leg	3-1-1	0
B2	Bent over dumbbell rows	4	10 each arm	3-1-1	0
B3	Swiss ball ab crunches	4	15	3-1-1	60 secs
C1	Burpees	10	30 secs	Fast!	90 secs

(Stretch)

EXERCISE GUIDE

Detailed demonstrations of the exercises are available to view through the Sculpt YouTube channel at **www.sculpt.me.uk**

EXERCISE 1: BODY WEIGHT SQUATS

Body parts worked: Legs, bottom, abs

- Stand upright with feet shoulder width apart.
- Squat back and down until thighs are parallel with the floor.
- Push yourself back up through your heels.

Progression:
- Add dumbbells held at shoulder level
- Increase weight to increase difficulty.

EXERCISE 2: KNEE PRESS-UPS

Body parts worked: Shoulders, chest, back of arms, abs

- With knees on the mat, place hands slightly wider than shoulder width apart.
- Engage ab muscles and lower your upper body to the floor by bending elbows.
- Push yourself back to starting position in a smooth motion.

Progression:
- Move knees further from hands.
- Take weight onto toes.

EXERCISE 3: PLANK

Body parts worked: Abs

- Facing downwards, take your weight on your elbows and toes, creating a bridge with your torso.
- Engage ab muscles and keep your back straight.
- Hold the position.

Progression:
- Try lifting an elbow/leg off the floor.
- Perform with elbows on a Swiss ball.

EXERCISE 4: HIGH STEP-UPS

Body parts worked: Legs, bottom

- Set up a step to around knee height.
- Place one foot on the step. Pushing through your heel, step up onto the box.
- Hold the position for a second and slowly control your step back onto the floor.

Progression:
- Add dumbbells.
- Increase the height of the step.

EXERCISE 5: UPRIGHT ROWS

Body parts worked: Upper back, biceps

- Set up a cable or resistance band and take both handles with arms extended, facing towards the anchor point.
- Pull the handles towards your chest, pulling your elbows back and squeezing your shoulder blades together.
- Hold the position for a second and slowly control the handles back to start position.

Progression: Increase weights or resistance of band.

EXERCISE 6: HIP BRIDGES

Body parts worked: Bottom, abs

- Lie on your back with your feet flat on the floor and knees bent.
- Push your hips towards the ceiling through your heels.
- At the top position, squeeze your bottom, pull in your abs, hold for a second and then slowly lower to the floor.

Progression: Perform exercise with feet on a Swiss ball.

EXERCISE 7: FAST STEP-UPS

Body parts worked: Cardio intervals

- Set up a step to around 20cm (8in).
- Perform fast alternating step-ups for the allotted time.

EXERCISE 8: DUMBBELL DEADLIFTS

Body parts worked: Legs, back, bottom, abs

- Stand upright with feet shoulder width apart and dumbbells held by your thighs.
- Engage your ab muscles and slowly bend forwards from the hips, keeping your head up and back very straight.
- Once the dumbbells reach your mid-thigh, start to bend your knees too.
- Go as deep as flexibility will allow and then push back up to standing through your heels, keeping back straight.

Progression: Increase weight to increase difficulty.

EXERCISE 9: DUMBBELL CHEST PRESS

Body parts worked: Shoulders, chest, back of arms, abs

- Take dumbbells in your hands and lie flat on your back on a bench or step with arms extended above your chest.
- Bring the dumbbells towards your chest by bending your elbows, keeping in line with your chest.
- Once elbows reach 90 degrees, push the weights back to their starting position.

Progression:
- Increase weight.
- Perform exercise on a Swiss ball.

EXERCISE 10: MOUNTAIN CLIMBERS

Body parts worked: Abs

- Facing the floor, take your weight on your hands and toes.
- Engage your ab muscles, keep your back straight.
- Alternately bring one knee towards your chest in a smooth, controlled motion.

Progression: Perform exercise with hands on a Swiss ball.

EXERCISE 11: WALKING LUNGES

Body parts worked: Legs, bottom

- Standing up straight, take a large step forwards with one leg to create a split stance.
- Bending your front knee to 90 degrees, bend your back knee in a controlled movement towards the floor.
- Keep your back straight and head up. Once your front thigh is parallel with the floor, push yourself back up to standing through your front heel.
- Repeat on the other leg in a 'walking' fashion.

Progression:
- Add dumbbells.
- Increase weight.

EXERCISE 12: DUMBBELL LAT PULL OVERS

Body parts worked: Upper back

- Take one dumbbell with both hands and lie flat on your back on a step or bench.
- Extend your arms straight above your chest and slightly bend your elbows.
- Slowly drop the dumbbell backwards until it reaches the top of your head.
- Hold the position for a second and then bring the dumbbell back to starting position.

Progression: Increase weight to increase difficulty.

EXERCISE 13: HEEL TAPS

Body parts worked: Abs

- Lie flat on your back on an exercise mat, taking both feet off the floor with knees bent to 90 degrees.
- Keeping your back flat, slowly lower one heel until it taps the floor and then bring it back to starting position.
- Repeat with the other leg.

Progression: Tap both heels at the same time to increase difficulty.

EXERCISE 14: DUMBBELL SQUAT-CURL PRESS

Body parts worked: Legs, bottom, arms, shoulders

- Stand with feet shoulder width apart and dumbbells held by your sides.
- Perform a squat. When back at the starting position, perform a bicep curl with the dumbbells and then lift them above your head until your arms are fully extended.
- Return to starting position.

  Progression: Increase weight to increase difficulty.

EXERCISE 15: BURPEES

Body parts worked: Cardio intervals

- Stand upright with feet shoulder width apart, bend over and place both hands on the floor in front of you.
- Kick both feet back behind you so your body is in a plank position with a straight back.
- Kick both feet back towards your hands and then jump up high off the floor and return to starting position.

EXERCISE 16: SINGLE ARM DUMBBELL ROWS

Body parts worked: Upper back, arms

- Set up a bench or step to around thigh height, take a dumbbell in one hand.
- With your right knee and right hand supporting you on the bench, straighten up your back and straighten out your left arm holding the dumbbell.
- Row the dumbbell towards your chest and armpit, bringing your elbow back.
- Return to starting position.

Progression: Increase weight to increase difficulty.

EXERCISE 17: COBRAS

Body parts worked: Back

- Lie on your front on an exercise mat and place your arms by your sides.
- Using your lower-back muscles, slowly raise your shoulders off the floor.
- At the top position, bring your arms off the floor and squeeze your shoulder blades together using your upper-back muscles.
- Return to starting position.

Progression: Perform exercise on a Swiss ball.

EXERCISE 18: BENT OVER DUMBBELL ROWS

Body parts worked: Upper back, arms

- Standing up straight, holding dumbbells by your sides, bend over into a deadlift, keeping your back straight.
- Extend your arms towards the floor, keeping your back straight and head up.
- Simultaneously row both dumbbells up towards your chest, squeezing your shoulder blades together.
- Return your arms to starting position.

Progression: Increase weight to increase difficulty.

EXERCISE 19: AB CRUNCHES

Body parts worked: Abs

- Lie flat on your back on an exercise mat.
- Put your hands to your temples and slowly lift your shoulders slightly from the floor using your abs.
- Return to starting position.

Progression: Perform exercise on a Swiss ball.

What to do next

If you have followed the 5:2 Bikini Diet and Sculpt 30 programme for four weeks, you should now see in the mirror a slimmer, leaner and healthier body. Congratulations – you have earned it! You should be proud that you have made a commitment to changing your body and health – but don't stop! Unfortunately, all results are reversible through inactivity, so visit the Sculpt website for an advanced online training programme, available at an exclusive 25 per cent discount in conjunction with *The 5:2 Bikini Diet*. Use code Sculpt52.

Yours in health,

David
www.sculpt.me.uk

CALORIE COUNTING REFERENCE

Food Type	cal per 100g/ml	pro (g)	carb (g)	fat (g)
Bread				
Breadcrumbs, manufactured	354	10.1	78.5	2.1
Brown bread	207	7.9	42.1	2
Brown, crusty	255	10.3	50.4	2.8
Brown, soft	236	9.9	44.8	3.2
Brown, toasted	272	10.4	56.5	2.1
Ciabatta	271	10.2	52	3.9
Currant bread	289	7.5	50.7	7.6
Garlic bread, prepacked, frozen	365	7.8	45	18.3
Granary	237	9.6	47.4	2.3
Granary, roll	238	10.2	42.7	4.2
Hamburger buns	264	9.1	48.8	5
Pitta, white	255	9.1	55.1	1.3
Tortillas, corn	222	6	47	3
White bread	219	7.9	46.1	1.6
White, crusty	262	9.2	54.9	2.2
White, soft	254	9.3	51.5	2.6
White, toasted	267	9.7	56.2	2
Wholemeal	217	9.4	42	2.5
Wholemeal, roll	244	10.4	46.1	3.3

Food Type	cal per 100g/ml	pro (g)	carb (g)	fat (g)
Wholemeal, toasted	255	11.2	49.2	2.9
Beans and Lentils				
Borlotti beans, canned and drained	53	4	6	1
Broad beans, raw	59	5.7	7.2	1
Cannellini beans, canned and drained	85	7.1	12.5	0.6
Chickpeas, canned and drained	115	7.2	16.1	2.9
Mixed beans, canned	100	6	15	1
Puy lentils, dried	297	24.3	48.8	1.9
Red kidney beans, canned and drained	100	6.9	17.8	0.6
Red lentils, split, dried	318	23.8	56.3	1.3
Breakfast Cereals				
Bran Flakes	330	10.2	71.2	2.5
Corn Flakes	376	7.9	89.6	0.9
Fruit 'n' Fibre	353	9	72.5	5
Muesli, Swiss style	363	9.8	72.2	5.9
Multi-Grain Start	369	7.9	85.2	3.5
Porridge with water	46	1.4	8.1	1.1
Porridge with whole milk	113	4.8	12.6	5.1
Special K	374	15	75	1.5
Weetabix	338	11.5	68.4	2
Condiments and Sauces				
Barbecue sauce	93	1	23.4	0.1
Brown sauce, sweet	98	1.2	22.2	0.1
Capers	14	1.4	1.3	0.3
Coconut milk, light	73	0.7	1.6	7
Green Thai curry paste	100	1.9	20	1.3
Harissa Paste	90	2.3	11.8	3.6

Food Type	cal per 100g/ml	pro (g)	carb (g)	fat (g)
Jerk paste	81	1.2	10	5
Miso soup paste	203	13.3	23.5	6.2
Olive paste	204	0.6	0.6	21.5
Peppers, pickled, sweet	34	1.8	7.1	0
Sweet chilli sauce	229	0.6	55.1	0.7
Tahini (sesame seed paste)	607	18.5	0.9	58.9
Tamarind paste	90	0.6	20.5	Tr
Tomato ketchup	115	1.6	28.6	0.1
Dressings				
Caesar dressing	542	2	3	58
Caesar dressing, light	109	3	12.5	6.2
French dressing	462	0.1	4.5	49.4
French dressing, fat free	38	0.1	9.9	0
Horseradish sauce	153	2.5	17.9	8.4
Light mayonnaise	288	1	8.2	28.1
Mayonnaise	691	1.1	1.7	75.6
Mirin (rice wine)	289	0.2	71.7	0.1
Nam pla (Thai fish sauce)	54	4.5	9	0.5
Salad cream	348	1.5	16.7	31
Salad cream, reduced fat	194	1	9.4	17.2
Mustards				
Dijon mustard	165	7.8	4.8	12
English mustard	160	8.2	18.7	5.6
Wholegrain mustard	140	8.2	4.2	10.2
Soy Sauce				
Dark soy sauce	75	6.2	10.9	0.5
Light soy sauce	52	2.5	10.5	trace
Stock cubes				
Chicken stock, made up per pack instructions	7	0.1	0.6	0.4

Food Type	cal per 100g/ml	pro (g)	carb (g)	fat (g)
Fish stock cube, made up per pack instructions	7	0.2	0.4	0.5
Vegetable stock cube, made up per pack instructions	10	0.1	0.5	0.6
Vinegars				
Balsamic vinegar	104	1.2	19.8	0
Cider vinegar	18	0	0.4	0
Red Wine vinegar	22	0.6	0.4	0
Rice vinegar	6	0.2	1.4	0
White wine vinegar	22	0	0.6	0
Worcestershire sauce	65	1.4	15.5	0.1
Dairy				
Butter, salted and unsalted	744	0.6	0.6	82.2
Cheddar, English	416	25.4	0.1	34.9
Cottage cheese, reduced fat	79	13.3	3.3	1.5
Cream cheese	439	3.1	Tr	47.4
Feta	250	15.6	1.5	20.2
Halloumi	315	22	0.8	24.6
Mozzarella	257	18.6	Tr	20.3
Parmesan	415	36.2	0.9	29.7
Roquefort	375	19.7	Tr	32.9
Skimmed milk	32	3.4	4.4	0.2
Yogurt, plain, low fat	56	4.8	7.4	1
Desserts and Puddings				
Sugar-free raspberry jelly	61	1.2	15.1	0
Drinks (alcoholic)				
Brandy	222	Tr	Tr	0
Lager (bottled)	29	0.2	1.5	Tr

Food Type	cal per 100g/ml	pro (g)	carb (g)	fat (g)
Red wine	68	0.1	1.5	0
Sherry, dry	116	0.2	1.4	0
White wine	66	0.1	0.6	0
Drinks (Non-alcoholic)				
Orange juice, unsweetened	36	0.5	8.8	0.1
Eggs				
raw, white	36	9	Tr	Tr
raw, whole	151	12.5	Tr	11.2
Flour and Baking				
Cocoa powder	312	18.5	11.5	21.7
Coconut, desiccated				
Cornflour	354	0.6	92	0.7
White breadmaking flour	341	11.5	75.3	1.4
White, plain flour	341	9.4	77.7	1.3
Yeast, dried	169	35.6	3.5	1.5
Fruit	35	0.3	8.9	0.1
Apples, cooking, peeled	47	0.4	11.8	0.1
Apples, eating, raw	95	1.2	23.2	0.3
Apricots, dried	188	4.8	43.4	0.7
Bananas, peeled	48	0.9	11.5	0.1
Cherries	37	0.9	8.7	0.1
Clementines, peeled	604	5.6	6.4	62
Grapes, black/white, seedless	60	0.4	15.4	0.1
Kiwi fruits	49	1.1	10.6	0.5
Lemons (whole)	19	1	3.2	0.3
Lime juice	9	0.4	1.6	0.1
Mangoes, peeled	57	0.7	14.1	0.2
Oranges, peeled	37	1.1	8.5	0.1
Peaches, flesh and skin	33	1	7.6	0.1

Food Type	cal per 100g/ml	pro (g)	carb (g)	fat (g)
Pears	40	0.3	10	0.1
Pineapples, canned in juice	47	0.3	12.2	Tr
Plums	36	0.6	8.8	0.1
Raisins	272	2.1	69.3	0.4
Raspberries, fresh	25	1.4	4.6	0.3
Strawberries	27	0.8	6	0.1
Herbs and Spices				
Basil, fresh	40	3.1	5.1	0.8
Cayenne pepper, ground	318	12	31.7	17.3
Coriander, fresh	20	2.4	1.8	0.6
Mint	43	3.8	5.3	0.7
Paprika powder	289	14.8	34.9	13
Parsley	34	3	27	1.3
Tarragon, fresh	49	3.4	6.3	1.1
Jams, Marmalades and Sweet Spreads				
Apricot jam	244	0.4	60.6	0
Blackcurrant jam	244	0.4	60.6	0
Honey	288	0.4	76.4	0
Marmalade	261	0.1	69.5	0
Peanut butter, crunchy	606	24	15	50
Peanut butter, smooth	607	22.8	13.1	51.8
Raspberry jam	244	0.5	60.4	0.1
Strawberry jam	244	0.4	60.6	0
Poultry				
Chicken breast, skinned and boned	148	32	0	2.2
Chicken breast, skinned and boned, stir-fried	161	29.7	0	4.6

Food Type	cal per 100g/ml	pro (g)	carb (g)	fat (g
Chicken, light and dark meat, roasted	177	27.3	0	7.!
Duck, meat only, roasted	195	25.3	0	10
Turkey mince, stewed	176	28.6	0	6
Turkey breast fillet, grilled	155	33	0	?
Fish and Seafood				
Anchovy fillets, canned in oil and drained	191	25.2	0	
Cod, raw	80	18.3	0	
Haddock fillets, raw	81	19	0	
Hake, raw	92	18	0	
Halibut, raw	92	17.7	0	
King prawns	74	16.3	0.5	
Monkfish, raw	66	15.7	0	
Prawns	99	22.6	0	
Salmon fillet, raw	180	20.2	0	
Scallops, frozen without shells	91	18.3	3.5	
Tiger prawns	65	14	0	
Trout, brown, raw	112	19.4	0	
Tuna steak, raw	136	23.7	0	
Tuna, canned in spring water and drained	105	25	0	
Pork/Ham				
Chipolata sausages, raw	275	13.9	3.	
Gammon, joint, boiled	204	23.3	(	
Ham, cooked, wafer thin	84	16.5		
Parma ham	223	27.2		
Pork loin chops, lean and fat, grilled	184	31.6		
Pork steaks, lean and fat, grilled	198	32.4		

Food Type	cal per 100g/ml	pro (g)	carb (g)	fat (g)
Spanish chorizo	291	18	3.2	23
Lamb				
Lamb breast, lean only, roasted	252	25.6	0	16.6
Lamb leg, lean only, roasted	203	29.7	0	9.4
Beef				
Bacon rashers, fat trimmed, grilled	214	25.7	0	12.3
Beef escalope (from fillet), raw	140	21.2	0	6.1
Beef mince, stewed	209	21.8	0	13.5
Beef rump steak, lean meat only, fried	183	30.9	0	6.6
Pastrami	123	19.4	1.8	4.3
Sausages, beef, grilled	278	13.3	13.1	19.5
Nuts and Seeds				
Almonds, blanched/flaked/ground	612	21.1	6.9	55.8
Cashew nuts, plain	573	17.7	18.1	48.2
Chestnuts, whole	170	2	36.6	2.7
Peanuts, plain	564	25.8	12.5	46
Pine nuts	688	14	4	68.6
Sunflower seeds	581	19.8	18.6	47.5
Walnuts, shelled	688	14.7	3.3	68.5
Oils and Fats				
Extra-virgin olive oil	899	0	0	99.8
Olive oil	899	Tr	0	99.9
Sesame oil	898	0.2	0	99.7
Sunflower oil, spray, light	522	Tr	Tr	55.2
Walnut oil	899	Tr	0	99.9
Pasta, Rice, Grains and Noodles				
Brown basmati rice	347	9.2	71.4	2.7

Food Type	cal per 100g/ml	pro (g)	carb (g)	fat (g)
Dry pasta, standard, raw	362	12	77	0.7
Dry pasta, wholewheat, raw	324	13.4	66.2	2.5
Egg noodles, boiled	62	2.2	13	0.5
Pearl barley, raw	360	7.9	83.6	1.7
Wholegrain rice	344	8	73	2.2
Sugar and Sweeteners				
Maple syrup	262	0	67.2	0.2
Dark brown sugar, soft	362	0.1	101.3	0
Sugar, granulated	400	0	100	0
Sugar, white	394	Tr	105	0
Sweets and chocolates				
Plain chocolate	510	5	63.5	28
Vegetables, raw				
Rocket leaves	25	0	2	0.6
Asparagus	25	2.9	2	0.6
Avocado pear	190	1.9	1.9	19.5
Beansprouts	31	2.9	4	0.5
Broccoli	33	4.4	1.8	0.9
Butternut squash	36	1.1	8.3	0.1
Cabbage, white	27	1.4	5	0.2
Carrots, old	35	0.6	7.9	0.3
Carrots, young	30	0.7	6	0.5
Cauliflower	34	3.6	3	0.9
Celery	7	0.5	0.9	0.2
Chillies, red	26	1.8	4.2	0.3
Courgettes	18	1.8	1.8	0.4
Cucumber	10	0.7	1.5	0.1
Garlic	98	7.9	16.3	0.6
Gem lettuce leaves	12	0.6	1.5	0.4
Ginger, root	49	1.7	9.5	0.7

Food Type	cal per 100g/ml	pro (g)	carb (g)	fat (g)
Green beans	24	1.9	3.2	0.5
Leeks	22	1.6	2.9	0.5
Lettuce	14	0.8	1.7	0.5
Mangetout	32	3.6	4.2	0.2
Mushrooms, chestnut	16	1.8	Tr	0.5
Mushrooms, common	13	1.8	0.4	0.5
Mushrooms, portobello	35	4	5	1
Mushrooms, shiitake, dried	296	9.6	63.9	1
Olives, black, pitted, in sunflower oil	466	0	20	40
Olives, green, pitted, in brine	103	0.9	Tr	11
Onions	36	1.2	7.9	0.2
Pak choi	19	1.5	2.2	0.2
Peas, frozen, raw	66	5.7	9.3	0.9
Potatoes, new	70	1.7	16.1	0.3
Potatoes, old	75	2.1	17.2	0.2
Red peppers (bell), stalks and seeds removed	32	1	6.4	0.4
Romaine lettuce heart	16	1	1.7	0.6
Shallots	20	1.5	3.3	0.2
Spinach	25	2.8	1.6	0.8
Spring onions	23	2	3	0.5
Swede	24	0.7	5	0.3
Sweet potato	87	1.2	21.3	0.3
Sweetcorn, on the cob	54	2	9.9	1
Tomato purée	76	5	14.2	0.3
Tomatoes	19	0.7	3.1	0.4
Tomatoes, canned	16	1	3	0.1
Tomatoes, cherry	23	1.2	3.3	0.6
Tomatoes, sun-dried	495	3.3	5.4	51.3